COSMETIC BLEPHAROPLASTY AND FACIAL REJUVENATION

SECOND EDITION

COSMETIC BLEPHAROPLASTY AND FACIAL REJUVENATION

SECOND EDITION

Stephen L. Bosniak, M.D., F.A.C.S.

New York Eye & Ear Infirmary
Manhattan Eye, Ear & Throat Hospital
New York, New York

Marian Cantisano Zilkha, M.D.

Center for Clinical Studies at Oftalmoclinica Botafogo,
Rio de Janeiro, Brazil
Total Rejuvenation Systems
New York, New York

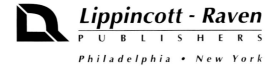

Lippincott - Raven
PUBLISHERS

Philadelphia • New York

Manufacturing Manager: Dennis Teston
Production Manager: Jodi Borgenicht
Production Editor: Elaine Verriest
Cover Designer: Patricia Gast
Indexer: Lynne Mahan
Compositor: Maryland Composition

Printed and bound in China

9 8 7 6 5 4 3 2 1

Library of Congress Cataloging-in-Publication Data

Bosniak, Stephen L.
    Cosmetic blepharoplasty and facial rejuvenation / Stephen L. Bosniak, Marian Cantisano
Zilkha.—2nd ed.
        p.   cm.
    Rev. ed. of: Cosmetic blepharoplasty. c1990.
    Includes bibliographical references and index.
    ISBN 0-397-58469-5 (hardcover)
    1. Blepharoplasty.   2. Surgery, Plastic.   3. Face—Surgery.   4. Rejuvenation.   I. Zilkha,
Marian Cantisano.   II. Bosniak, Stephen L.   Cosmetic blepharoplasty.   III. Title.
    [DNLM: 1. Blepharoplasty—methods.   2. Face—surgery.   3. Reconstructive Surgical
Procedures.   4. Rejuvenation.   WW 205 B743c 1998]
    RD119.5.E94B67   1998
    617.7'710592—dc21
    DNLM/DLC
    for Library of Congress   98-7633
                                                                                  CIP

To our parents, Samuel and Thelma Bosniak
Dr. Luiz and Duca Cantisano,
the future Dr. Raiane Cantisano

Contents

Contributing Authors

Gregory Chernoff, M.D., F.R.C.S. (C) *Assistant Clinical Professor, Indiana University; Laser Skin Care Salons International, Inc.; and Chernoff Plastic Surgery and Laser Center, 9002 North Meridian Street, Suite 205, Indianapolis, Indiana 46260*

Steven B. Hopping, M.D., F.A.C.S. *Associate Professor of Surgery, George Washington University Hospital, Washington, D.C. and Director, The Center for Cosmetic Surgery, 1145 19th Street NW, Suite 707, Washington, D.C. 20036*

Preface to the First Edition

At first glance, cosmetic blepharoplasty may appear to be an easily performed procedure. It is, however, fraught with complexities that, if unrecognized, may lead to inadequate results and unhappy patients.

Cosmetic Blepharoplasty has been conceived as a complete guide to cosmetic eyelid surgery. Based on a comparison of normal anatomy and involutional changes, a methodical approach to corrective surgery is presented. Corrective and functional improvement is the goal.

I sincerely hope that the detailed preoperative evaluation of the patient, the outline of surgical options, intraoperative insights, and descriptions of recommended procedures will allow the cosmetic blepharoplasty surgeon to achieve satisfactory cosmesis without compromise of eyelid function.

Stephen Bosniak, M.D., F.A.C.S.

Preface to the First Edition

Preface

Since the publication of *Cosmetic Blepharoplasty* in 1990, the application of advanced technology—most notably the refinement of carbon dioxide laser and endoscopic technology, the recognition of pre- and postoperative skin therapies—has significantly enhanced the quality of the result of cosmetic blepharoplasty. Rather than merely performing a blepharoplasty, the procedure has truly become a "Total Eyelid Rejuvenation." Upper lid myocutaneous resections, levator aponeurotic repair, lipocontouring, and preseptal skin resurfacing rejuvenate the upper lid from within and without. Transconjunctival lower lid lipocontouring with lateral canthal plication and suspension return a youthful level and contour to the lax lower lid, providing a secure, well-positioned lid that will support a resurfaced anterior lamella.

Periocular support and rejuvenation are prerequisites for successful blepharoplasty. Full face rejuvenation procedures complement cosmetic periocular surgery. And whether performed by the same surgeon or another, they can conveniently be offered simultaneously.

Internally supported brows (via transblepharoplasty or endoscopic fixation) can provide appropriate brow level and contour that is augmented with forehead resurfacing. Full face resurfacing, facial lipocontouring, and lipoaugmentation can be supplemented with injectable autogenous collagen and fibroblasts as well as synthetic injectable gels and can ameliorate residual contour irregularities. Immobilizing dynamic rhytids with Botox allows for more effective resurfacing in the glabellar, crow's feet, and forehead areas. Residual furrows can be augmented with a variety of filling agents. These nonincisional, noninvasive techniques can also be applied to ear lobe and nasal recontouring with dramatic results.

However, the carbon dioxide laser is not magic. The effectiveness of the instrumentation requires a new aesthetic and does not eliminate the need for mastery of basic surgical principles. This instrument does not transform a poor surgeon into a better one. Quite the contrary, only the accomplished aesthetic surgeon can realize the true potential of this technology and avoid the complications of its misuse.

Radiosurgery continues to have many advantages over cold steel, and may be an efficient intermediary step in learning the use of the carbon dioxide laser as an incisional tool. The Erbium-Yag, Krypton Diode, and Nd:YAG lasers, as well as flashlamp technology, show promise in the future of facial rejuvenation.

It is our sincere hope that cosmetic surgeons will find this volume useful in their evaluation of potential candidates and in their surgical approach to these patients.

Stephen Bosniak, M.D., F.A.C.S.
Marian Cantisano Zilkha, M.D.

Acknowledgments

We would like to thank our patients who have consented to having their photos reproduced in this volume and who continue to be an inspiration. We would also like to thank Bill Bernstein, Ana Lucia Caldas, Coherent Medical, Con Bio Inc., Ellman International, Lavinia Errico, Dr. Alphonso Fatorelli, Maria Theresa Fatorelli, Dr. Jon Garito, Dr. Greta Hanna, Dr. Stephen Lore, Karen Luhman, Dr. Miguel Padilha, Irlacy Rodrigues, Cees Penning, and Dr. Alan Engler for their cooperation and assistance and Craig Luce for his artistic insight and expert illustrations. Our special thanks to Joan and Dan Sabatino for their tireless preparation of this manuscript.

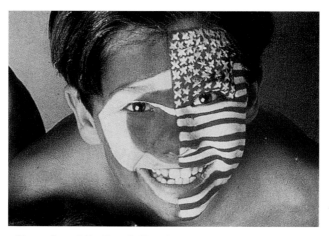

(From Jornal Do Brasil "Domingo" magazine June, 1997)

CHAPTER 1

Introduction

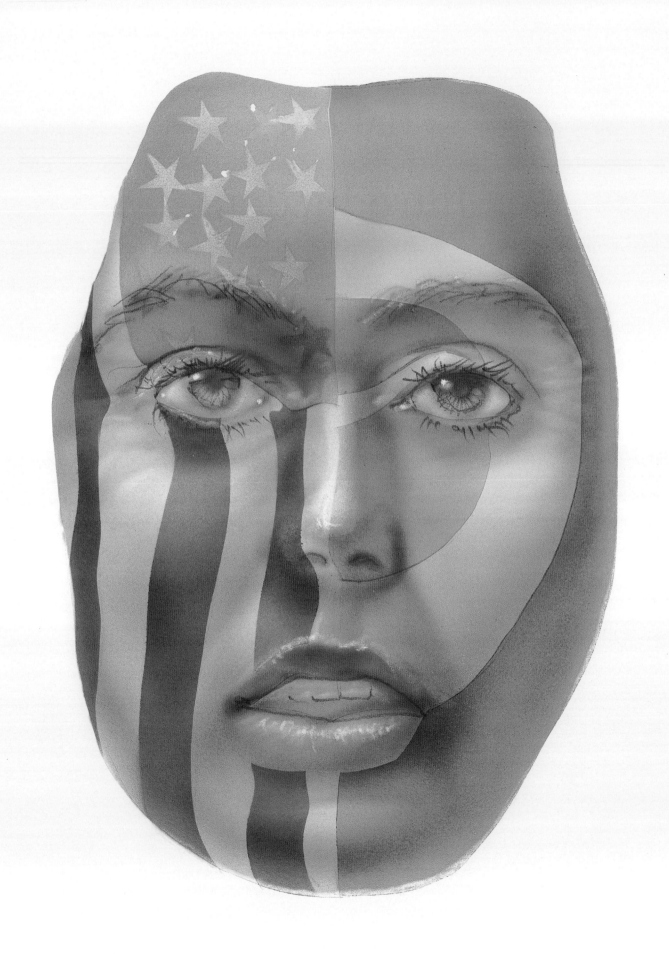

PATIENT SELECTION

The motivation of patients requesting cosmetic blepharoplasty may be obscure or apparent. Patients with specific complaints about their appearance and a clear realization of the limitations of surgery are ideal surgical candidates (Figs. 1A,B, 2A,B). Although patients' trust in the surgeon is a crucial factor in the patient–surgeon relationship, patients with vague complaints who do not involve themselves in the decision-making process, who simply say, ''Make me look better. Do whatever you have to do, I trust you,'' may have unrealistic expectations and may not be happy with the surgical outcome, no matter how technically perfect it may be. It is surgeons' responsibility to themselves and their patients to determine what physically objectionable parameters they can correct. To this end, sitting down with a patient, a recent photograph or Polaroid photograph taken during this initial consultation, and a mirror are the minimum prerequisites for patient satisfaction after cosmetic eyelid surgery. If the patient is uncertain about which findings are objectionable, a reversed mirror will provide additional details. It forces the patient to look at his or her face as the world sees it, and not as he or she is accustomed to seeing it. Computer-generated imaging may dramatically illustrate the proposed improvements in eyelid and facial features; however, the image produced must not be interpreted as a guarantee of the surgical result. Reviewing old photographs of patients is also helpful in tailoring the procedure to them. This discussion will emphasize to patients that each procedure is unique (Figs. 3A,B, 4A,B, 5A,B, 6A,B).

A second consultation before surgery may be necessary, when the patient and the surgeon can review a series of detailed preoperative medical photographs and/or computer-generated images. The development of rapport and the establishment of an uninhibited mode of communication are essential. The surgeon and the patient can scrutinize each detail in question. The patient can specify which deformities are unwanted, and the surgeon can then suggest which are amenable to surgical revision. If the surgeon is unable to identify the source of the patient's complaint, remedy is impossible. The surgeon must translate the patient's subjective complaint into an objective physical finding. Technical perfection is not a guarantee of patient satisfaction. The patient must have realistic expectations of what the outcome of surgery can be and must be aware of the limitations of surgery.

Patients also must be aware of the variability in healing and the essential differences in the turgor and texture of each person's skin. They should be informed that everyone heals differently and that the healing process may take longer on one side of the face than on the other. The patient and the surgeon must decide what is most appropriate for the patient, what alterations in eyelid contour are most compatible with the face, and what general facial alterations the patient would like to consider concomitantly. Often, subtlety is very effective, and the postoperative result is not too jarring. Friends and family may comment on how rested the patient looks and not be struck with the fact that the patient had surgery (Figs. 7A,B, 8A,B). A well executed blepharoplasty can change the appearance of the entire face. Patients may want to see how they will look after blepharoplasty, before deciding whether they want additional facial surgery. Mature patients older than seven decades with borderline tear films and marginal corneal compensation may be much happier with conservative upper eyelid resections that minimize the risk of postoperative lagophthalmos and corneal exposure and avoid the annoyance of a potentially dry eye. Conservative upper lid myocutaneous resections combined with laser resurfacing will beautifully recontour the upper lid without risk of lid retraction, lid lag, or lagophthalmos. The transconjunctival approach to lower lid blepharoplasty will minimize the possibility of lower lid retraction and disturbance of the tear film (Fig. 9A,B).

Patients must understand that although they will look better and feel better about themselves, they cannot expect

(text continues on page 7)

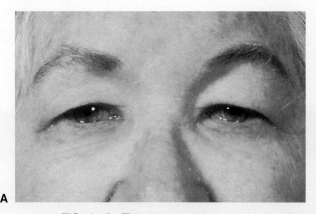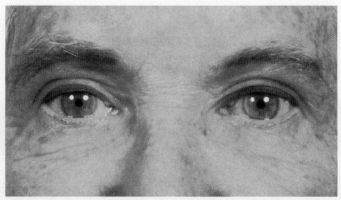

FIG. 1. A: This 70-year-old woman's chronic blepharitis was caused by marked redundancy of the upper lid folds. **B:** Following an upper lid blepharoplasty, her facial appearance was greatly improved, and she no longer suffered from chronic blepharitis.

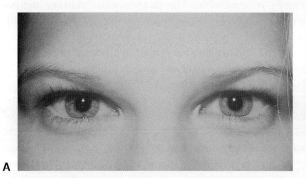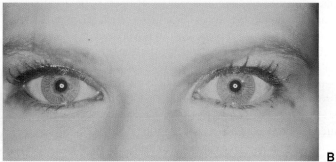

FIG. 2. A: This 22-year-old model was worried about her heavy upper lids and her lower lid contours. **B:** Without a radical change in her appearance, her eyes have become more striking after sculpting of her brow fat pockets and plicating her lateral canthi.

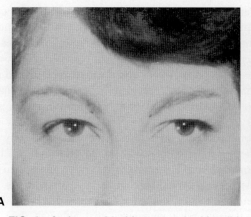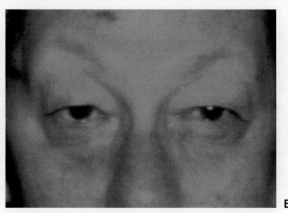

FIG. 3. A: At age 21, this woman had low lid crease–fold complexes and full superior sulci. **B:** At age 73, even with brow elevation, her palpebral apertures have narrowed, and her upper lid lashes are completely hidden by her upper lid folds.

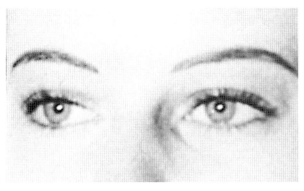 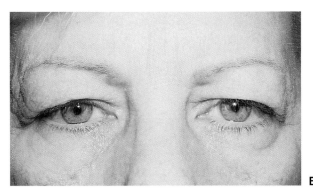

A   B

FIG. 4. A: At age 18, this young woman had well formed lid crease–fold complexes. **B:** 45 years later, her upper lid folds rest on her lashes, her upper lid creases are almost completely hidden, and her superior sulci are full.

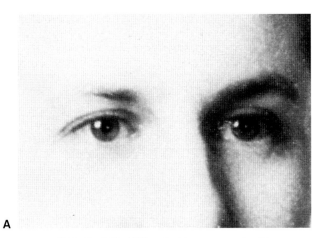 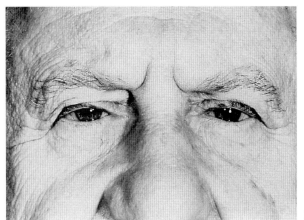

A   B

FIG. 5. A,B: Without skin care and with more exposure to the environment, in the past men often aged more dramatically than women. The lower, flatter, heavier brow descends more quickly than a woman's.

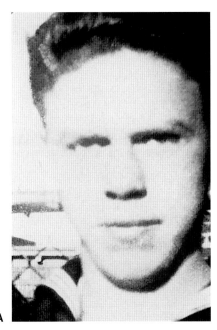 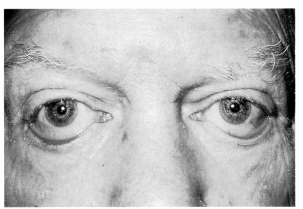

A   B

FIG. 6. A,B: Sun exposure for the sensitive patient may evoke not only rhytid formation but also cicatricial retraction of the lower lids and cutaneous carcinoma formation.

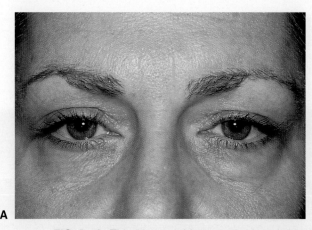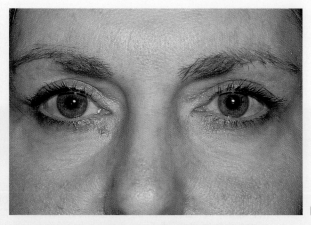

FIG. 7. A: This 39-year-old woman had moderate upper lid fold fullness with brow fat pocket thickening and moderate lower lid fat herniation. **B:** Following upper lid myocutaneous resections, lipocontouring with suborbicularis brow fat sculpting, and lower lid transconjunctival lipocontouring, she appears well rested.

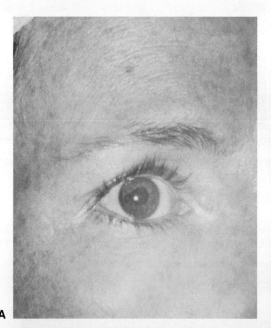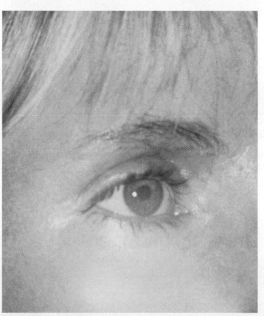

FIG. 8. A: This 33-year-old woman had moderate upper lid fullness and mild lower lid fatty prolapse. **B:** Her lid contours are strikingly improved with upper lid and brow contouring, lower lid transconjunctival lipocontouring, and eyelid resurfacing.

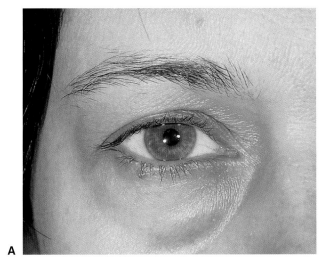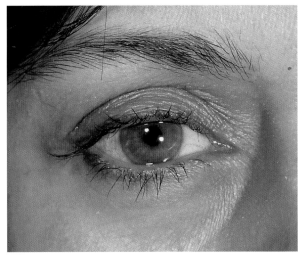

FIG. 9. A,B: Conservative upper lid myocutaneous resections with lipocontouring and lower lid transconjunctival lipocontouring can rejuvenate the eyelids without disturbing the palpebral aperture or tear film.

their lives to change dramatically. Expecting cosmetic surgery to change one's lifestyle and psyche is simply unrealistic. Blepharoplasty patients should not necessarily expect to look younger; they can expect to look more alert and healthy and less weary. However, adding resurfacing to the surgical menu will certainly rejuvenate the face (Fig. 10A,B).

Since keloid formation at the sites of eyelid incisions is exceptionally rare, dark-skinned patients with a history of keloid formation can expect excellent results following blepharoplasty (Fig. 11A,B). At the lateral orbital rim, the thin eyelid skin becomes thicker facial skin; therefore, temporal extensions of the lid incisions beyond the lateral orbital rim

are to be avoided, if possible, since they may be subject to hypertrophy and keloid formation. Direct brow elevations should be discouraged in patients with a history of keloid formation. Cutaneous hypertrophic scars may melt with cautious subcutaneous injections of methylprednisolone acetate (Depo-Medrol). These injections may cause skin atrophy and pigmentary disturbances. Black patients must accept the remote but plausible possibility of postoperative postinflammatory hyperpigmentation, which in most cases resolves completely within several months of surgery, or hypopigmentation.

Asian patients are also excellent candidates for blepharoplasty. The patient–surgeon dialogue, however, must in-

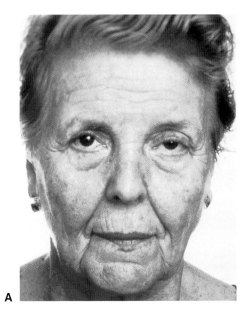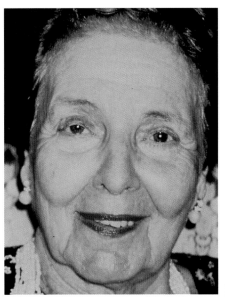

FIG. 10. A,B: This 82-year-old woman noted a marked improvement following correction of left upper lid ptosis, transconjunctival lower lid blepharoplasty, and light full-face CO_2 laser resurfacing.

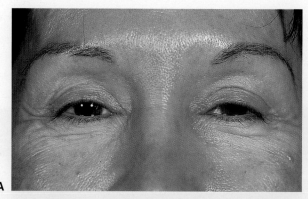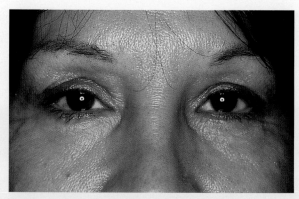

FIG. 11. A,B: This 38-year-old Middle Eastern woman had an excellent result following bilateral ptosis correction, lateral canthoplasties, transconjunctival blepharoplasties, and Botox injections to the crow's-feet.

clude a discussion of lid-crease height, depth, and contour. Asian patients must realize that cosmetic blepharoplasty may occidentalize their appearance if a high lid-crease incision is made. Asian patients are also at risk for cutaneous pigmentary disturbances and keloid formation; the same cautions apply as in black patients.

Since the introduction, acceptance, and proven effectiveness of carbon dioxide (CO_2) laser resurfacing and, more recently, of erbium:yttrium-aluminum-garnet (Er:YAG) laser resurfacing, the criteria for patient selection have expanded. Static facial rhytids and irregularities of facial skin texture and pigmentation have become appropriate deformities amenable to correction. The dynamic rhytids of the forehead, glabella, and lateral periorbital areas can be addressed with injections of botulinum toxin type A purified neurotoxin complex (Botox) followed by CO_2 laser resurfacing. Consideration of skin texture, pigmentation, and actinic damage has new relevance (Fig. 12A–F).

A convenient classification for preoperative evaluation is: fair skin, Mediterranean skin, Asian skin, and black skin. Patients with darkly pigmented skin may not be ideal candidates. In patients who are very dark, preoperative test laser applications and follow-up observations will be helpful. In the majority of these patients, pretreatment before laser resurfacing, lighter CO_2 laser application or Er:YAG laser resurfacing, careful postoperative follow-up and treatment will give the desired result.

PATIENT PREPARATION

Surgeons must deal with the unpleasant but important task of preparing patients for the unwanted and the unexpected. They must somehow inform them without frightening them unnecessarily. Even though the likelihood of serious complications is remote if the right care is taken, surgeons must forcefully describe the potential complications of this surgery without completely dissuading patients from the procedure. Patients will undoubtedly forget the

many complications discussed and may not be able to recount this discussion accurately in the event of a postoperative complication. They may, however, recall that complications were discussed, even if the specifics of the discourse are forgotten. Patients must be informed of the potential pitfalls of the surgery—at least the generalized possibilities of bleeding, infection, and scarring. For informed consent, the most serious complications must be discussed. The preparation must be complete and all-inclusive to be of value. However, giving patients a list of potential complications or a tape recording or videotape of the discussion may be overwhelming for them. The exceedingly rare but nonetheless devastating complications of visual disturbance and even death should not be omitted from a preoperative discussion of potential complications. The specific abnormalities of lid level and contour, lid closure dysfunction, and tear film aberrations should also be discussed (Table 1). Even though CO_2 laser blepharoplasty has

TABLE 1. *Potential complications of cosmetic eyelid surgery (preoperative discussion with patient)*

Death
Visual disturbance or decreased vision
Dry eyes
Red eyes
Failure to close eyelids
Asymmetry of eyelids
Drooping of one or both upper lids
Pulling down of lower lids
Eyelids open too wide (staring look)
Excessive tearing
Blockage of tear ducts
Double vision
Restriction of movement of one or both eyes
Discolored eyelids
Numbness of eyelids
Decreased blinking
Small lines or cysts on eyelids, milia
Residual skin excess
Residual fat pockets

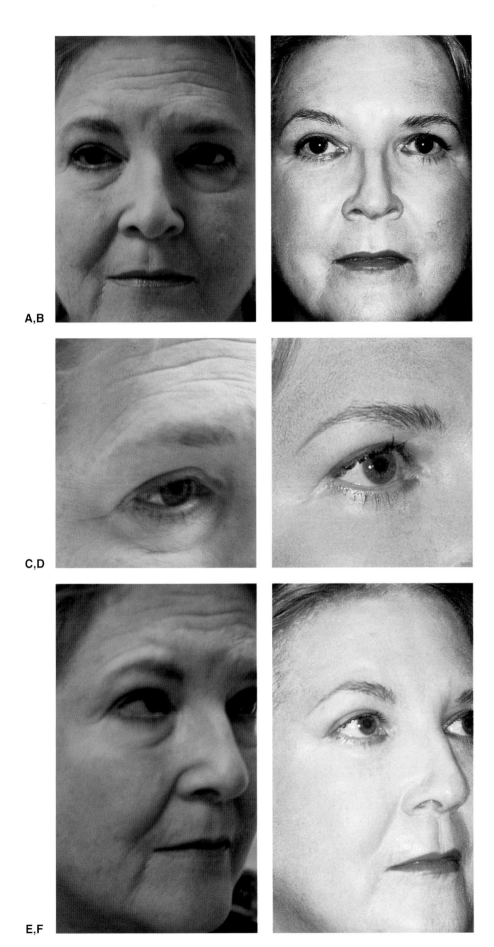

A,B

C,D

E,F

FIG. 12. A–F: This 45-year-old woman had moderate upper lid and brow heaviness, moderate lower lid fatty prolapse, moderate brow and glabellar furrowing, and moderate deepening of the nasolabial folds. She had striking improvement of her eyelid and facial contours following CO_2 laser upper lid and brow lipocontouring, transconjunctival lower lid lipocontouring, glabellar and forehead Botox injections, and full-face CO_2 laser resurfacing followed by hyaluronic acid gel [e.g., Hylaform (Biomatrix, Saint Tropez, France), Restylane (Q Med, Uppsala, Sweden)] injections to her nasolabial folds.

greatly reduced the possibility of intraoperative and postoperative bleeding, as well as augmenting the accuracy of lipocontouring, the general discussion of potential complications remains the same. There is no substitute for good surgeon–patient rapport and well informed patients.

Preoperative discussions with patients having laser facial rejuvenation must familiarize them with the normal landmarks of the postoperative recovery period. The areas covered with dressings should remain without discomfort and remain covered for 5 to 10 days; they will require little care. The areas of the face not covered will feel tight and warm and may have a ''burning'' feeling; they will require cleansing and constant lubrication. Patients can expect a considerable amount of secretions during the first 3 days accompanied by crusting in areas that are not lubricated frequently enough. After 5 days, any residual crusting should be minimal. We usually replace dressings as needed until day 10. This is followed by a period of general erythema that may vary in intensity from mild (in darker-complected patients) to marked (in fair-complected patients) and that will vary in duration, usually from 4 to 12 weeks. After postoperative week 2, this can be covered with makeup without difficulty. Between the second and third postoperative weeks, patients may experience facial itching, which, if not controlled, may lead to transient excoriations. Between the third and fourth postoperative weeks, darkly pigmented patients may experience transient hyperpigmentation that lasts 3 to 12 weeks. This hyperpigmentation can be alleviated with topical fading creams and alpha-hydroxy acid (AHA) peels.

The potential complications of laser facial rejuvenation include prolonged erythema, dyspigmentation, scarring due to secondary infections (bacterial, herpetic, and fungal), and heightened response to laser energy and excessive laser applications. The possibility of dyspigmentation can be minimized by pretreating darkly pigmented patients and performing a test-patch application on those at risk for pigmentary disturbances. Bacterial and herpetic infections should be treated prophylactically. Patients who smoke, have had phenol peels, or have taken isotretinoin (Accutane) during the year preceding the laser resurfacing may not be candidates for laser facial rejuvenation. We prefer to resurface cautiously, telling patients that we can always do more later (Table 2).

Although not as critical when CO_2 laser incisional blepharoplasty techniques are used to facilitate intraoperative hemostasis and minimize postoperative oozing and subcutaneous ecchymosis, it is essential for patients to avoid aspirin, aspirin-containing compounds (Table 3), and cigarette smoking for at least 2 weeks preoperatively. During the preoperative months, reducing the quantity of cigarettes smoked or eliminating them completely also will facilitate wound healing and decrease postoperative edema.

Most patients can benefit from a home care program of AHA peels that also contain bleaching agents. This program should begin at least 2 weeks preoperatively and be supplemented with weekly glycolic acid peels. This preparation is particularly helpful for patients having facial resurfacing.

Patients with multiple periocular comedones or inclusion cysts should undergo a rigorous skin cleansing program beginning 6 to 8 weeks preoperatively. Facial cleansing systems and treatments appear to enhance skin turgor, resilience, and pliability. Patients applying topical tretinoin (Retin-A) cream to the face and eyelids should continue until the day of surgery. The long-term effects of chronic alcohol intake—multiple telangiectases and altered blood coagulability—cannot be altered or reversed with short-term abstinence, but should be noted.

TABLE 2. *Potential complications of laser facial rejuvenation*

Prolonged erythema
Pigmentary abnormality
Surface irregularities
Primary cutaneous scarring
Cutaneous scarring secondary to skin infection
Eyelid malposition
Reactivation of herpetic infection
Demarcation lines

TABLE 3. *Preoperative notice to patients*

For 2 weeks before your surgery, do not take any medications that contain aspirin as an ingredient. Please check the labels of any medications you take (even those available without a prescription) to see that you do not take aspirin. Taking aspirin will tend to increase your tendency to bleed at the time of surgery.

This is a partial list of the more common aspirin-containing products:

Alka Seltzer	Doan's Extra Strength Analgesic
Anacin	Dristan
APC	Empirin
ASA	Emprazil
Ascriptin	Equagesic
Asodeen	Excedrin
Aspergum	Fiorinal
Aspirin	Four Way Cold Tablets
Backache Caplets	Midol
Bufferin	Motrin
Cephalgesic	Naprosyn
Cheracol Caps	Nobaxisal
Children's aspirin	Percodan
Cope	Phenaphen
Coricidin	Trigesic
Darvon compound	Vanquish
Darvon with ASA	Zactrim
Darvo-Tran	

Other anticoagulants, antiparkinsonism medications, and monoamine oxidase inhibitors must also be discontinued preoperatively. Cardiac and antihypertensive medications should be continued until the time of surgery after clearance by your physician.

Anticoagulant therapy should be discontinued 2 weeks before surgery to avoid persistent clotting abnormalities during surgery. Monoamine oxidase (MAO) inhibitors also should be discontinued 2 weeks before surgery to avoid complicating drug interactions at the time of surgery. Diuretic, antihypertensive, antiglaucoma, and cardiac medications should be continued with medical monitoring until the time of surgery. Patients taking such medications should be seen and cleared by their internists before surgery.

Patients should be psychologically prepared for their postoperative course. No matter how benign the surgeon views a patient's recovery, he or she should not forget that most patients have not undergone this type of surgery before and have not seen what a blepharoplasty patient looks like during the first postoperative days. It is helpful to tell patients that they will not look good for the first week following surgery. Even though CO_2 laser incisional techniques and the lower lid transconjunctival approach have virtually eliminated ecchymosis in most patients, some lid edema may persist for weeks. Pre- and postoperative lymphatic drainage massage (manual or mechanical) will alleviate this (Fig. 13A–C).

Even with absolute hemostasis at the termination of the surgical procedure, patients should expect what they will view as marked edema. The edema will subside rapidly during the next week, although its complete resolution may take 4 to 6 weeks, especially when orbital fat has been removed. There is the rare instance of postblepharoplasty lymphedema that may take months to resolve. Erythema at the incision sites will fade rapidly from scarlet, to red, to pink over several weeks, but again complete blending of the incision may take months. Although in most cases there is no ecchymosis after lower lid transconjunctival laser blepharoplasty, subcutaneous ecchymosis, when it occurs, is at first localized; it will then lighten and spread inferiorly over the malar eminence and often into the cheeks. This may take 3 to 4 weeks to vanish completely. Conjunctival chemosis may follow transconjunctival lower lid lipocontouring and lateral canthal suspension. A more rapid alleviation of all of the above transient maladies is accomplished with lymphatic drainage massage.

Patients will see improvement within the first week after surgery. The improvement will become more marked as the edema subsides. However, if there is a residual contour irregularity, it cannot be assessed until 6 to 8 weeks postoperatively.

In addition to postoperative iced-compress applications for 72 hours, various pharmacologic, homeopathic, and para-

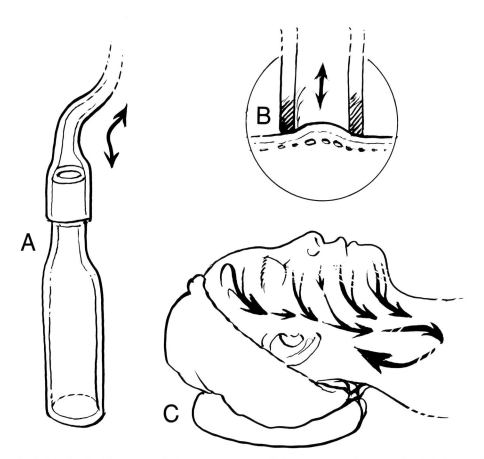

FIG. 13. A–C: Mechanical lymphatic drainage massage utilizing gentle suction can stimulate lymphatic flow and reduce postoperative edema. (Lymphobiology, developed by Catherine Atzen, San Jose, Calif)

medical adjuncts instituted preoperatively have been suggested to decrease the severity and duration of postoperative edema. These include the following:

- Dexamethasone sodium phosphate (e.g., Decadron) 8 mg intramuscularly the night before surgery, 8 mg intravenously (i.v.) before the first incision at the time of surgery, and 8 mg i.v. immediately after surgery, followed by an oral dexamethasone dose pack tapered over 6 days.
- Arnica sublingual pellets, three the night before surgery, three on the morning of surgery and then every 2 hours while awake on the evening following surgery and the next 2 days.
- Preoperative and postoperative lymphatic drainage massage.

In our hands, the use of CO_2 laser incisional techniques and lymphatic drainage massage have significantly reduced postoperative edema and obviated the use of perioperative dexamethasone.

A transient superficial numbness of the upper eyelid may occur secondary to resection of the subcutaneous fascia and its sensory nerve endings, but it should resolve within 6 to 8 weeks after surgery. Lower lid anesthesia does not occur with the transconjunctival approach. Fair-skinned patients with fine telangiectatic upper lid pretarsal vessels may note that the vessels and a slightly erythematous flush are visible and persist after surgery. Fine-wire radiosurgical ablation or krypton laser application can ameliorate these.

The treatment of lower lid dark circles has improved during the last several years. Patients may confuse lower lid bags with lower lid hyperpigmentation, and the two components must be evaluated individually. Treatment with hydroquinone and/or glycolic acid bleaching creams, supplemented with glycolic acid peels, can yield great improvement in most patients (Fig. 14A,B). If prolapsing lower lid orbital fat casts a shadow, accentuating lower lid dark circles, transconjunctival lipocontouring will further improve the appearance of the lid. In addition, Er:YAG and/or CO_2 laser resurfacing will even lower-lid skin texture and pigmentation.

PREOPERATIVE MEDICAL EVALUATION

Patients' safety and well-being are of paramount importance. Although the surgeon should always be cognizant of medical expenditures and should eliminate unnecessary testing, the preoperative workup should not be compromised if there is any doubt about patients' medical status. Not every operation demands a full laboratory workup. The obvious necessity of establishing patients' cardiopulmonary stability, general health, and blood clotting status is further reinforced by the need to be certain that they are not afflicted with specific ailments that may directly affect the surgical outcome (Table 4).

Chronically boggy upper and lower lids with secondary dermatochalasis and lichenification of the skin may be the result of thyroid dysfunction (usually myxedema), renal disease, incipient congestive heart failure, a hyperallergic state, or localized topical allergy. Prolapsed orbital fat or ptotic lacrimal glands may be sequelae of a hyperactive thyroid or Sjörgen's disease. Resection of lid tissue in these patients may be a frustrating experience for both surgeon and patient if the underlying medical condition is not first stabilized. Recurrent myxedema or lid infiltration will cause recurrence of lid dysfunction and contour irregularities. Biopsy of bilaterally prolapsed orbital lobes of the lacrimal glands may be appropriate if sarcoidosis is suspected.

Young patients, usually females in their 20s and 30s, with a history of bilateral or unilateral lid swelling may have true blepharochalasis, a syndrome of unknown etiology associated with intermittent eyelid edema. These patients should be informed that their edematous episodes may continue and may result in gradual stretching of the lid skin requiring additional procedures in the future. This should be differentiated from dermatochalasis (redundancy of the upper eyelid fold unassociated with lid edema),

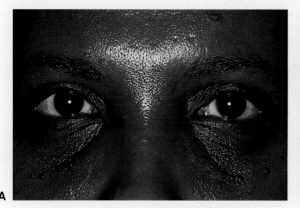
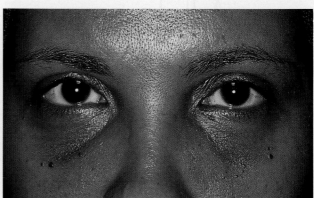

A   B

FIG. 14. A,B: This 46-year-old black-skinned woman with marked lower lid dyspigmentation responded well to bleaching creams, alpha-hydroxy acid peels, and CO_2 laser resurfacing.

TABLE 4. *Eyelid malpositions and possible systemic causes*

Swollen eyelids
    Thyroid dysfunction (hyper- or hypo-)
    Renal disease
    Cardiovascular disease
    Allergy
    True blepharochalasis
    Dacryoadenitis
Narrowed palpebral apertures
    Ptosis
    Myasthenia gravis
    Dermatochalasis
    Orbital tumor
    Enlarged or ptotic lacrimal glands
Inferior scleral show
    Normal anatomic variant
    Axial myopia
    Shallow orbits
    Thyroid lid retraction
    Retrobulbar mass

TABLE 5. *Preoperative workup*

Current photographs
    Full face, both eyes together, each eye separately (front and side views). Appropriate lighting and positioning are essential. For proper orientation, the base of the nose should be on the same horizontal plane as the tragus. Any head or chin depression or elevation will mask the true palpebral aperture.
Old photographs
    To establish the longevity of palpebral aperture asymmetry
Complete blood cell count in patients over 40 years or with history of anemia. Prothrombin time, partial thromboplastin time, and platelet count in patients with history of easy bruising or bleeding disorder.
Electrolytes and SMA 12 in patients over 60 years or with history of hypertension.
Triiodothyronine (T_3) and thyroxine (T_4) if any doubt about thyroid status; if surgeon's index of suspicion for thyroid dysfunction is marked, a more complete endocrinologic workup is indicated.
Electrocardiogram on every patient over 60 years
Chest x-ray if there is any history of pulmonary disease

which is usually an inherited trait or gradually acquired and secondary to cutaneous elastotic degeneration.

Acquired narrowing of the palpebral apertures without obvious levator aponeurotic disinsertions and with associated compromise of levator excursion would indicate the need for a myasthenia gravis workup (electromyography with or without edrophonium chloride testing). Systemic myasthenia gravis will require therapy, but systemic medication for ocular myasthenia gravis may not necessarily eliminate the need for eyelid surgery. An acquired mechanical ptosis with reduced levator excursion may also be secondary to a lid or orbital mass.

Acquired inferior scleral show may be related to hyperthyroid lid retraction and should be distinguished from congenitally shallow orbits, axial myopia, retrobulbar tumors, or a normal variant of eyelid anatomy. Old photographs will distinguish between acute and long-standing changes, even if patients and their families are not able to provide pertinent history.

Exophthalmometry (Naugle or Hertel) will distinguish lid proptosis from lid retraction, but orbital computed tomography may be necessary to distinguish monocular thyroid lid retraction and proptosis from an orbital tumor (Table 5).

Preoperative ophthalmologic examination is essential to document visual acuity, peripheral visual fields, intraocular pressure, tear film stability, tear quantitation (baseline tear function), strength of lid closure, lagophthalmos, and symmetry of palpebral apertures. The surgeon must communicate with the examining ophthalmologist to ensure that the necessary tests are performed. The preexistence of dry eyes, keratitis sicca, residual facial palsy, lid lag, or lagophthalmos from previous cosmetic surgery or postoperative ptosis from previous cataract, glaucoma, or retina surgery will

have a definite bearing on the extent of lid resections proposed, as well as on the associated procedures offered by the eyelid surgeon.

PREOPERATIVE MEASUREMENTS AND OBSERVATIONS

Table 6 lists preoperative measurements. Table 7 compares the idealized eyelids and palpebral apertures with the involutionally changed periocular structures.

Age-related changes in skin texture and turgor, as well as loss of subcutaneous support, in conjunction with environmental skin changes yield an altered appearance of the

TABLE 6. *Preoperative measurements and observations*

Vertical palpebral aperture
Horizontal palpebral aperture
Inferior scleral show
Distance of lid crease from lid margin
Direction and angle of upper lid lashes
Level and contours of brows, with special note of level of superior orbital rim
Level and angle of lateral canthi
Depth and symmetry of superior sulci
Lid contour irregularities (discrete or confluent convexities or concavities), with special attention to superior nasal and inferior lateral fat pockets
Location of inferior orbital rim and relationship to skin excess or fat prolapse
Lid margin malposition
Lower lid horizontal laxity
Canthal tendon laxity
Punctal position

TABLE 7. *Normal periocular anatomic relationships and contrasting involutional changes*

	Normal/idealized	Involutional changes
Brow	At or above superior orbital rim Gentle arch highest at junction of temporal one-third and nasal two-thirds	Below level of superior orbital rim Flattened arch
Superior sulcus	Flat	Excessively deep (fat atrophy) Excessively full (skin redundancy)
Vertical palpebral aperture	10 mm	Decreased (ptosis) Increased (inferior scleral show or upper lid retraction)
Upper lid crease	8–10 mm above lashes	Elevated (levator aponeurotic disinsertion) Obliterated (redundant lid fold)
Upper lid fold	Mild draping over crease	Excessive (obliterating crease) Retracted into superior sulcus (levator disinsertion)
Horizontal palpebral aperture	34 mm	Narrowed with canthal tendon laxity
Lateral canthal angle	Acute	Rounded with canthal tendon laxity or dehiscence
Lower lid margin	At or above inferior limbus	Inferior scleral show
Punctal position	Not visible; in lacrimal lake	Vertically directed or everted

eyelids and facial structures and a displacement of the periocular tissues. The flaccid tissue cannot resist gravity, and everything heads south. The brows may become ptotic, descending below the superior orbital rim in women, losing their arch, and in men drooping to a level precariously close to the upper lid lashes. This inferior brow displacement causes a secondary redundancy of the upper lid fold. Resecting or resurfacing the upper eye skin without first elevating or supporting the eyebrow will be ineffective if there is associated brow ptosis.

If the levator aponeurosis is disinserted, as evidenced by an elevated lid crease–fold complex and a deep superior sulcus with normal levator excursions, it must be advanced and repaired during the upper lid blepharoplasty before li-

pocontouring and myocutaneous resection are performed (Fig. 15A,B).

Before the lower lid can be resurfaced, laxity of the lid margin and lateral canthal tendon must be corrected. The angle of the lateral canthus and the apposition of the lid margin to the globe must also be restored before the lower lid anterior lamella is treated.

Rejuvenation of the eyelids is most prominently about restoration of function and not simply about aesthetics.

Vertical Palpebral Aperture

Measuring the distance between the upper and lower lid margins will reveal the presence of a true ptosis. The av-

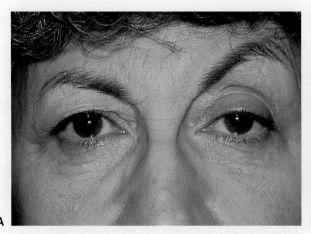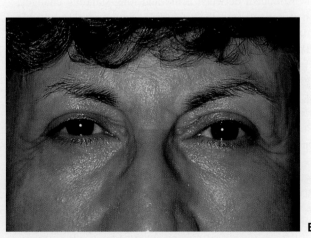

A

B

FIG. 15. A: This 66-year-old woman demonstrates an obvious left upper lid ptosis with an elevated lid crease–fold complex and secondary left brow elevation. **B:** Following correction of the left upper lid ptosis with levator aponeurotic advancement and bilateral upper lid blepharoplasty, she has palpebral aperture, upper lid, and brow symmetry.

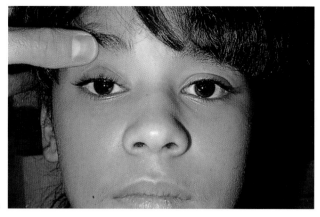
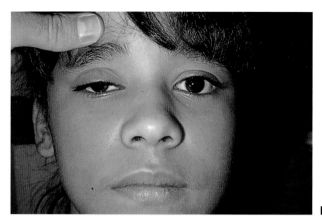

A   B

FIG. 16. A: Elevating the brow can widen the palpebral aperture and reduce blepharoptosis. **B:** Depressing the brow can narrow the palpebral aperture and accentuate ptosis.

erage vertical palpebral aperture is approximately 10 mm, with the upper lid margin 1 to 2 mm below the superior limbus and the lower lid margin at the level of the inferior limbus. The brow should be held in its normal position at the superior orbital rim while the vertical palpebral aperture is measured using a clear plastic ruler so that the eye may be visualized during the measurement. Raising or depressing the brow will camouflage or accentuate ptosis (Fig. 16A,B) and upper lid fold redundancy (Fig. 17A,B). A markedly redundant upper lid fold may obscure the superior lid margin and may have to be lifted gently for accurate quantitation of the palpebral aperture. A patient with an obvious ptosis may have a vertical palpebral aperture of 10 mm or greater if there is inferior scleral show.

Horizontal Palpebral Aperture

The average horizontal palpebral aperture in an adult is 30 to 34 mm. Laxity or dehiscence of the medial or lateral canthal tendons will cause distortion and narrowing of the horizontal palpebral aperture. Marked lower lid ectropion without canthal tendon laxity will cause gross distortion of the lower lid margin but may not shorten the horizontal distance between the canthal angles. However, horizontal wedge or inverted pentagonal resections of the lower lid margin without prior correction of concomitant canthal ten-

don laxity will yield narrowing of the horizontal palpebral aperture.

Inferior Scleral Show

Inferior scleral show is the distance from the inferior limbus to the lower lid margin. It may occur normally as an anatomic variant without sequelae, or it may be the result of senescence (lid margin and canthal tendon laxity) , hyperactive thyroid–induced lid retraction, high myopia, shallow orbits, or a hypoplastic inferior orbital rim.

We feel that there is rarely an indication for the transcutaneous approach for the lower lid. Subciliary incisions, even without lower lid skin or myocutaneous resections, cause lower lid retraction to some degree. In patients with preexisting scleral show, a transcutaneous lower lid blepharoplasty is contraindicated. In these patients, lower lid laser resurfacing of the pretarsal skin should be avoided.

Horizontal resections of the lax lower lids also may exaggerate inferior scleral show. If the lower lid is resting on the convex inferior surface of the globe, tightening the lid may pull it further inferiorly. These patients need superiorly directed support, recession of lower lid retractors, and canthal tendon plication in addition to lid margin tightening (Fig. 18A,B).

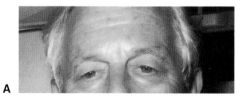
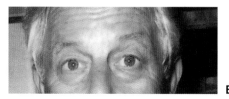

A   B

FIG. 17. A: Brow ptosis can accentuate lid fold redundancy. **B:** Brow elevation will reduce lid fold excess.

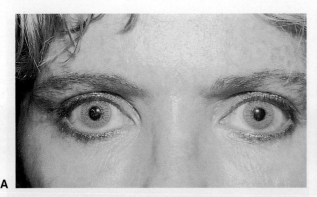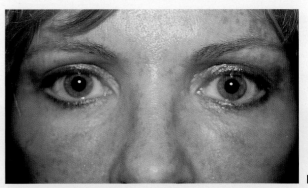

FIG. 18. A: This 42-year-old woman was referred to us for correction of lower lid retraction following transcutaneous lower lid blepharoplasty. **B:** She was considerably improved following recession of her lower lid retractors and lateral canthal plication.

Distance of Upper Lid Crease to Lid Margin

This is the distance of the anterior expansions of the levator aponeurosis to the lid margin. Retraction of these adhesions from the pretarsal orbicularis muscle and skin accompanies the retraction of a dehisced or rarefied levator aponeurosis. The hallmark of involutional aponeurotic dehiscences is an elevated lid crease (see Fig. 15A,B).

Upper Lid Lashes

The normal gentle upward sloping of the upper lid lashes may be altered with levator aponeurotic disinsertions. Mechanical ptosis or pseudoptosis secondary to marked excess of upper lid skin weighing down the upper lid and resting on the lashes may cause these lashes to become more inferiorly directed. Repair of the levator aponeurotic disinsertion, resection of excessive skin and orbicularis muscle, formation of an adequate lid crease, or a necessary combination of these will properly redirect the upper lid lashes.

Superior Sulcus

The idealized flat contour of the female superior sulcus may be distorted by prolapsed fat pockets or redundant skin. It may be completely hidden by a ptotic brow drooping below the superior orbital rim. Recontouring the superior sulcus will often be the primary objective of blepharoplasty. The male brow and superior sulcus, although still amenable to cosmetic surgery, do not lend themselves to the same recontouring as does the female brow–sulcus complex. The male superior sulcus is full, at least in part because the brow is flatter, with less arch. Patients with ptosis and levator aponeurotic disinsertions may have deep, flat superior sulci. They might find their ptosis objectionable but like their superior sulcus contours. Reapproximations of the dehisced aponeurosis to the tarsus without skin, orbicularis muscle, and fat resection will correct their ptosis but change the contour of their superior sulcus. This usually

will not make patients happy. Similarly, preoperative asymmetry of the superior sulci should alert the surgeon to the likelihood of levator aponeurotic disinsertion and ptosis or unilateral brow ptosis (see Fig. 15A,B).

Involutional orbital fat atrophy and sunken superior sulci may also be objectionable to patients. This deformity is more difficult to correct. Autogenous fat transfer may be associated with an irregular contour and atrophy. Rigid synthetic methyl methacrylate implants have been wired to the superior orbital rim with some success in anophthalmic patients. Autogenous dermis fat grafts are bulky and have also been used with variable success in the correction of superior sulcus deformities in anophthalmic patients.

Brows

Most female patients like their brows above the level of the superior orbital rim, with a gentle arch reaching its highest point at the junction of the nasal two-thirds and the temporal one-third (approximately in line with the temporal limbus). Historically, the female brow is usually plucked to conform to the idealized contour: fullest nasally as far medially as the medial orbital rim, tapering temporally, and exposing a bare expanse over the temporal superior orbital rim. This nonsurgical recontouring may make accurate brow assessment difficult. The surgeon should ask patients where the brows were before plucking, examine old photographs, and look for traces of remaining brow follicles. Plucking may satisfactorily camouflage minimal brow ptosis and contour irregularities, if there is no secondary displacement of lid tissues.

The male brow is thicker, flatter, and less well defined, with less arch or no arch at all (see Fig. 5A,B). It may be tempting for the surgeon to elevate the male brow slightly to facilitate deepening of the superior sulcus, but this often is inappropriate for the male physiognomy and should be approached with caution. However, temporal brow ptosis with secondary hooding of the upper lid is not uncommon and can be corrected conveniently and effectively with a direct temporal brow resection or internal suspension and forehead laser resurfacing.

Suborbicularis Brow Fat Pocket

Patients with heavy upper lids, a full superior sulcus, and a thick upper lid fold that obscures the upper lid crease require sculpting of the suborbicularis brow fat pocket (see Fig. 7A,B). In these patients, resecting or vaporizing preaponeurotic fat alone may not create enough definition of the superior sulcus. Internal brow suspension may easily be performed after sculpting the brow fat pocket.

Lateral Canthal Angle

The conjoined tendons of the upper and lower lids form an acute angle. In the average non-Asian patient, the lateral canthus is slightly superior to the medial canthus. Any rounding or inferior displacement of the lateral canthus will be cosmetically significant. Lower lid cicatricial deformities secondary to aggressive skin resections, phenol peels, or excessive resurfacing can cause rounding of the lateral canthus. Bilaterally rounded lateral canthi should alert the surgeon that previous cosmetic surgery may have been performed. The lateral canthal angle can be reconstructed after release of any cicatricial adhesions. Lateral and inferolateral displacements of the lateral canthi may also be manifesta-

tions of congenital euryblepharon or a variant malformation.

Routine blepharoplasty techniques can be altered to accommodate these deformities.

Lid Surface Contour Irregularities

Lid irregularities secondary to prolapsed orbital fat abutting orbicularis muscle and skin are dome-shaped and smooth. Each fat pad may yield a discrete mass (two in the upper lid and three in the lower lid). They may appear as a confluent mass in the lower lid or be undifferentiated and incorporated into a redundant fold of the upper lid. Herniated fat pads can be further identified by gentle pressure on the globe. Pressure on the globe via the upper lid will accentuate the inferior pockets. Qualitative and quantitative assessment of these inferior fat pockets is facilitated by observing them in all fields of gaze. Inferior pockets are accentuated with supraduction. Abduction accentuates the nasal pocket, and adduction accentuates the temporal pocket (Fig. 19A–C). Pressure applied inferiorly will accentuate the superior pockets. A preoperative drawing delineating these fat pockets will be most useful intraoperatively when subcutaneous infiltration of the lids and patients' supine position cause a coalescing of the lid surface contours. The superior fat pockets are most apparent nasal to the superior punctum and temporally.

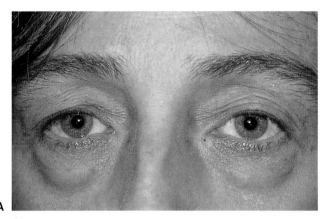

A

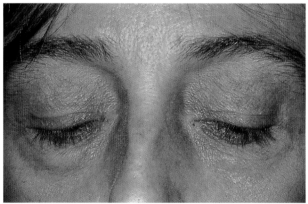

B

C

FIG. 19. A: Prolapsed inferior orbital fat pockets are visualized in the primary position. B: The inferior fat pockets are retracted on downward gaze. C: The inferior pockets are accentuated on upward gaze.

Careful demarcation of the nasal pocket is essential, since it is often medial to the nasal border of the upper lid incision and therefore not completely exposed during lid dissection. The skin–muscle flap must either be extended or retracted to effectively expose these pockets without enlarging the incision. The inferior fat pockets are typically larger than the superior pockets. Careful preoperative annotation of the lateral extent and contour of the temporal fat pocket is necessary, since a lateral extension of the conjunctival incision may be necessary to expose this pocket.

Skin rhytids and excess folds and surface irregularities are effectively addressed with resurfacing techniques rather than additional skin resection.

Hypertrophic Orbicularis Muscle

The position and contour of hypertrophic pretarsal orbicularis muscle differ from those of orbital fat. Hypertrophic orbicularis muscle most commonly occurs as a transverse ridge or band on the anterior tarsal surface extending as far inferiorly as the inferior tarsal border (see Fig. 2A,B). It may be associated with deep smile creases and definitely is accentuated by smiling, obliterating any fatty convexities. The muscle is semilunar and draped, is not at all dome-shaped, is not segmental, and extends horizontally over the entire width of the lid (Fig. 20A,B). Hypertrophic preseptal orbicularis muscle of the upper lid, although not as well defined, can contribute bulk to the upper lid fold and may be resected during blepharoplasty.

Inferior Orbital Rim

The inferior orbital rim is a useful landmark to palpate when patients considering lower lid blepharoplasty are examined. Prolapsed fat and redundant folds may be part of a malar bag and not amenable to standard lower lid approaches. In cases of mild malar cutaneous redundancy, la-

ser resurfacing can be used effectively. More prominent malar deformities will require direct resection and secondary resurfacing. Facial skin distal to the orbital rims is thicker than eyelid skin and must be treated differently. This also is very apparent at the lateral orbital rim and in the brow (Fig. 21). Hypoplastic or flat inferior orbital rims may require malar augmentation (Fig. 22A,B).

Lid Margin Malpositions

Involutional entropion and ectropion of the lower lid can be corrected concomitantly with lower lid blepharoplasty.

Punctal Position

The punctum is normally not visible without retracting the lower lid. It is hidden nasally in the lacrimal lake in close apposition to the globe. If the punctum can be seen without touching the lid, it is considered everted. Lower lid skin resection or pretarsal laser resurfacing anterior to the punctum will accentuate punctal eversion. Postoperative punctal eversion, even without frank ectropion, will cause epiphora and an unhappy patient.

Canthal Tendon Laxity

Lid margin laxity is determined by grasping the lid and pulling it away from the globe. If it can be retracted 6 mm or more from the globe, it is deemed lax. At the same time, if nasal traction on the lid narrows the horizontal palpebral aperture, the lateral canthal tendon is lax. If lateral traction on the lid displaces the punctum temporally, the medial canthal tendon is lax. Tightening a lax canthal tendon must precede horizontal shortening of the lid margin to avoid distortions of the horizontal palpebral aperture.

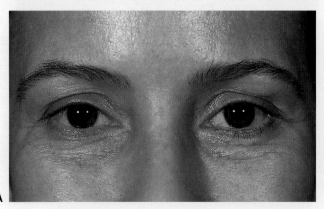 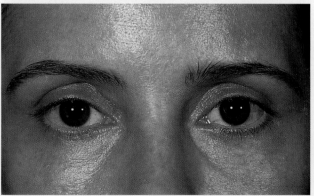

A   B

FIG. 20. A: This 39-year-old woman had thick brow fat pockets, moderate lower lid hypertrophic orbicularis muscles, and mild lower lid fatty prolapse. **B:** Her appearance is improved after upper lid suborbicularis brow fat resection and lower lid lipocontouring with lateral canthal and orbicularis muscle suspension.

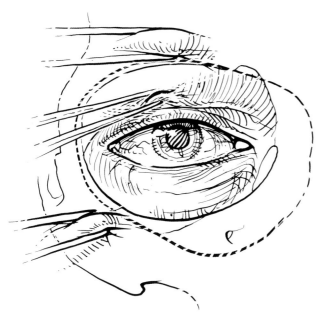

FIG. 21. The orbital rims are the demarcation lines between thin eyelid skin and thicker facial, brow, and forehead skin.

SURGICAL PLANNING

Performing Multiple Procedures Concomitantly

Each of the following procedures can be performed singly or in combination with others. Obviously, in tailoring a procedure to suit patients, the surgeon can use a variety of techniques. There is, however, a general scheme to follow (Fig. 23A–F). The brow level must be determined and fixed before the upper lid resections can be demarcated. Upper lid skin resection before the brows are elevated may result in marked lagophthalmos and a greatly reduced distance between the eyebrows and the eyelashes. Many surgeons prefer to operate on the upper lids before operating on the lower lids. There is no rigid rule that demands that upper lid skin resection be performed before lower lid blepharoplasty dissection. In fact, if the surgeon thinks that the lower lids will be more difficult to correct, he or she may want to perform the lower lid dissection first. Lower lid margin and canthal tendon laxity must be corrected before lower lid resurfacing. If lateral canthal surgery is proposed, the upper lid wounds should be left open temporally over the lateral orbital rim to visualize placement of the supporting suture.

Facial rejuvenation including operating on the brows and the upper and lower lids at one sitting provides an avenue of efficiency. It leaves additional time for vasoconstriction and hemostasis as the surgeon operates on the contralateral brow or lid. CO_2 laser incisional techniques further enhance intraoperative efficiency by providing improved hemostasis.

The following is an effective order of procedures: With the patient in the upright position, the appropriate brow elevation and contour are determined and marked. While the brow is held in position, the upper lid resection is demarcated. The patient is put in the supine position and se-

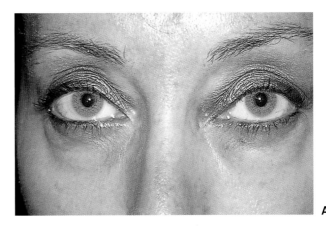

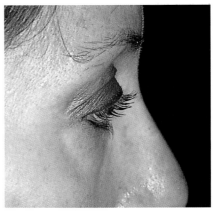

FIG. 22. A: These prolapsed inferior fat pockets are clearly superior to the inferior orbital rim. **B:** Viewing the prolapsed fat pockets from the side, in addition to palpating the inferior orbital rim, differentiates orbital fat from malar bags or festoons. This patient demonstrates hypoplastic inferior orbital rims.

dated. In the right upper lid, subcutaneous infiltration is performed. Supraorbital and supratrochlear regional blocks are given. The right brow is infiltrated. The left upper lid and brow are infiltrated and blocked. A right transcutaneous infraorbital regional block is given and then supplemented with subconjunctival infiltration. The left lower lid is then blocked and infiltrated.

The right upper lid myocutaneous resection is performed with the 0.2-mm UltraPulse handpiece (Coherent Medical, Palo Alto, Calif) or a 50-mm Silk Touch handpiece (Sharplan Lasers, Allendale, NJ). The CO_2 laser is used for all incisions, dissections, resections, and vaporization. A myocutaneous flap is developed superiorly, exposing the orbital septum and the superior orbital rim. The orbital septum is opened. The prolapsed orbital fat is transected over a moistened cotton-tipped applicator. The residual fat is vaporized. The superior orbital rim is exposed. The right brow fat pocket is resected, and the brow is internally supported with 4-0 Prolene sutures. The left upper lid and brow are addressed.

(*text continues on page 22*)

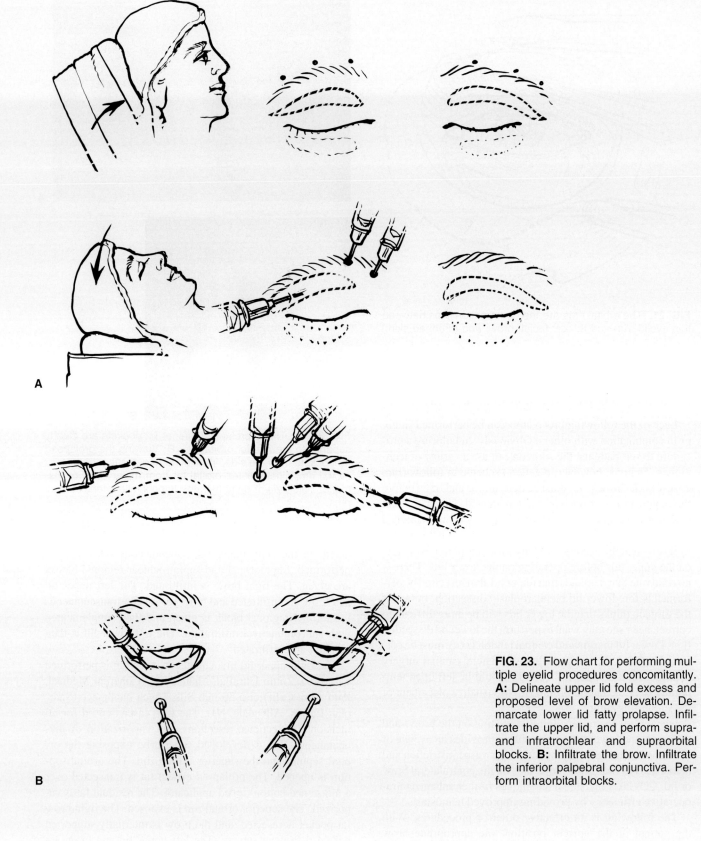

FIG. 23. Flow chart for performing multiple eyelid procedures concomitantly. **A:** Delineate upper lid fold excess and proposed level of brow elevation. Demarcate lower lid fatty prolapse. Infiltrate the upper lid, and perform supra- and infratrochlear and supraorbital blocks. **B:** Infiltrate the brow. Infiltrate the inferior palpebral conjunctiva. Perform intraorbital blocks.

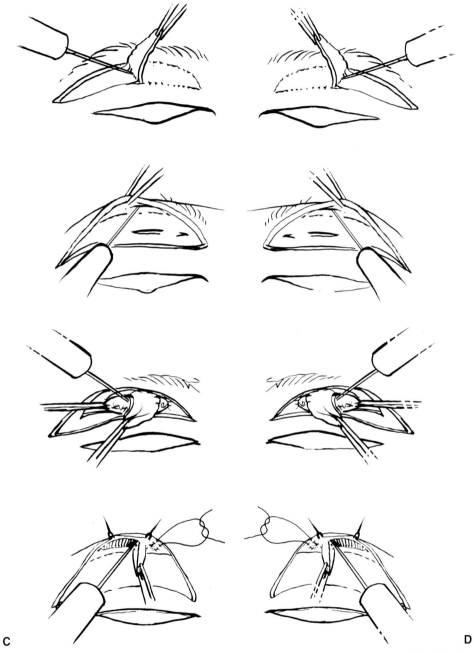

C   D

FIG. 23. *Continued.* **C,D:** The upper lids are resected, the fat is sculpted, the suborbicularis brow fat sculpted, and the brow internally supported.

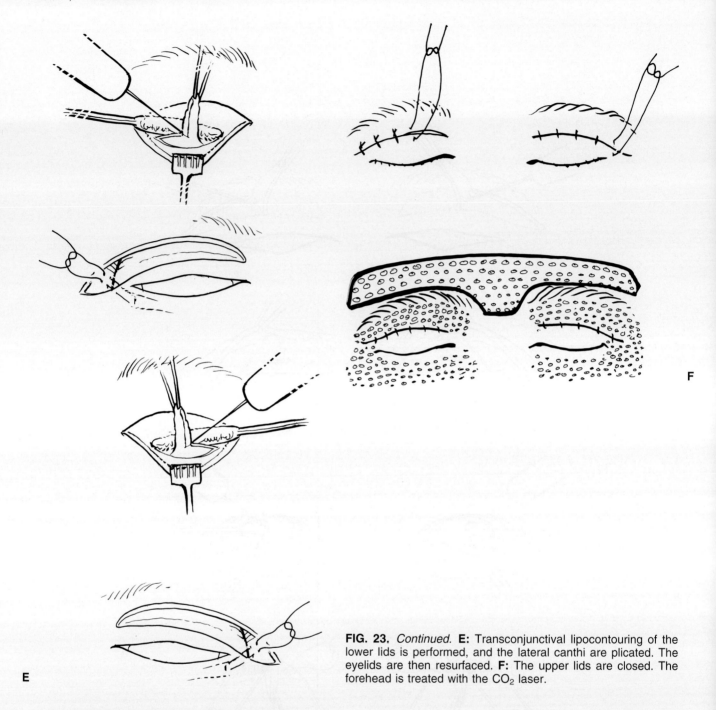

FIG. 23. *Continued.* **E:** Transconjunctival lipocontouring of the lower lids is performed, and the lateral canthi are plicated. The eyelids are then resurfaced. **F:** The upper lids are closed. The forehead is treated with the CO_2 laser.

A right lower lid transconjunctival blepharoplasty is performed. A right lateral canthal tendon plication is performed. A left lower lid transconjunctival blepharoplasty is performed. A left lateral canthal tendon plication is performed. The right upper lid incision is sutured; then the left upper lid is closed.

A 3 cm strip of forehead just above the brow and the eyelids are resurfaced.

Anesthesia

Intravenous sedation makes the experience of surgical eyelid rejuvenation more pleasant for patients. It eases any discomfort associated with local infiltration of the eyelids. In the past, resection of orbital fat pockets was painful and often produced traction on the extraocular muscles, with resultant bradycardia or even asystole, adding emphasis to the need for constant patient monitoring. However, the use of the CO_2 laser for fat vaporization has markedly reduced orbital traction and discomfort. Some systemic sedation, an analgesic or amnestic agent, or a combination of these is definitely helpful. Tranquilizing patients before they are transported to the operating room promotes a feeling of well-being and further allays any anxiety. Surgeon–patient rapport enhances patient tranquility nonpharmacologically.

A thorough preoperative therapeutic drug history is im-

TABLE 8A. *Medications to be discontinued preoperatively (partial list)*

Antiparkinsonism medications
Aspirin (2 weeks preoperatively)
Warfarin (Coumadin) (2 weeks preoperatively)
Monoamine oxidase inhibitors (2 weeks preoperatively)
Phenothiazines
Butyrophenones

portant. Certain medications must be continued up to the time of surgery, whereas others should be discontinued. Diuretics may cause hypokalemia. Although the medications may be continued, any serum potassium abnormalities must be corrected. Topical and systemic beta-blocking agent therapy also should be continued, but the possibility of cardiac decompensation and bronchoconstriction exists. Tricyclic antidepressants should be continued, with the anesthesiologist watching for possible hypertension, hypotension, and tachycardia. It is important to continue antihypertensive therapy, including a morning dose for afternoon cases. MAO inhibitors should be discontinued at least 2 weeks before surgery because hypertensive crises have been described when MAO inhibitors have been taken concomitantly with opioids or sympathomimetic amines. If a patient is taking antiparkinsonism therapy, the phenothiazines (e.g., chlorpromazine [Thorazine]) and the butyrophenones (e.g., droperidol [Inapsine]) should be avoided (Table 8A). Although the majority of patients having surgery in an office-based operating room setting do not need preoperative medication, some of the commonly used effective preoperative medications include meperidine (Demerol), diazepam (Valium), and lorazepam (Ativan) (Table 8B).

All eyelid procedures can be performed in a well equipped office operating suite. Many can be performed with straight local anesthesia. For procedures lasting more than a half hour and with patients over 60 years of age, we prefer to have an anesthesiologist participate. Call it "twi-

light," "fractional," "MIS" (monitored intravenous sedation), "MAC" (monitored anesthetic control), or "narcoleptic" anesthesia, there is no question that it is safer to have an anesthesiologist monitoring patients' blood pressure, pulse, electrocardiogram, and pulse oximetry while intravenous medication is being given.

Neuroleptanalgesia is defined as the production of a state of psychic indifference to stimuli. It consists of titrated and monitored intravenous administration of different drugs to achieve varying degrees of sedation, amnesia, or attenuation of response to stress. The patient is sedated and then operated on after local anesthetic infiltration.

The dose of narcoleptic or neuroleptanalgesic anesthesia can be titrated effectively at the surgeon's request when more or less patient cooperation is needed. During the surgery, the surgeon's attention and the nursing staff's attention are focused entirely on the operative field. Having qualified medical personnel whose sole function is to monitor the patient's blood pressure and cardiopulmonary status and to treat any untoward medical events can only increase the margin of patient safety and comfort. Suggested "cocktails" vary from institution to institution and from anesthesiologist to anesthesiologist, and they are modified from patient to patient. Our basic requirements are the following: We want patients awake for any skin demarcation. We want them sleeping for the infiltration. We want them comfortably sedated for the dissection, and we want them awake for final skin trimming and levator aponeurotic reapproximation. Manipulating the orbital fat with clamping, cutting, and cauterizing may require additional sedation, since traction is applied on the deeper orbital tissues with this technique and can be uncomfortable. CO_2 laser fat resection and vaporization and radiosurgical fat resection reduce orbital manipulation and discomfort but are also facilitated with sedation. Obviously, a combination of long-acting and short-acting agents may be required during the procedure, depending on its length.

Once a patient is comfortably premedicated, a short-act-

TABLE 8B. *Drugs used for premedication*

Drug	Usual dose and route[a]	Remarks
Meperidine (Demerol)	25–75 mg i.m.	Less potency, intermediate duration, and fewer cardiovascular effects make it narcotic of choice in elderly
Diazepam (Valium)	5–10 mg p.o.	Good tranquilizer; good amnesic; not analgesic or antiemetic; painful when given i.m.
Lorazepam (Ativan)	2 mg p.o.	Similar to diazepam but more profound amnesia and longer duration, which can be problem in elderly and ambulatory patients
Phenothiazines (e.g., promethazine [Phenergan])	12.5–25 mg i.m.	Neuroleptics; good antiemetics; patients may exhibit extrapyramidal movements; should be avoided in patients on antiparkinsonism therapy; may cause hypotension
Hydroxyzine (e.g., Vistaril)	25–100 mg p.o.	Antihistamine; good anxiolytic; good antiemetic; potentiates narcotics; painful when given i.m.

[a] Elderly patients often require reduced doses. When in doubt, premedication should be decreased. Supplemental sedation can be given intravenously in the operating room if needed.

Modified from Konovitch JW. Anesthetic management of the aging patient. In: Bosniak S, ed. *Advances in ophthalmic plastic and reconstructive surgery, vol II. The aging face.* Elmsford, NY: Pergamon Press, 1983;307–308; with permission.

TABLE 9A. *Neuroleptanalgesia*

Drug[a]	Usual dose and route	Remarks
Fentanyl (Sublimaze)	0.002 mg/kg i.v.	Potent synthetic narcotic; rapid onset; can cause significant respiratory depression; can cause bradycardia; cardiovascular stability if adequate ventilation; poor sedative
Droperidol (Inapsine)	0.1 mm/kg i.v.	Butyrophenone; rapid onset with reasonably short duration but relatively long half-life; accumulates and outlasts fentanyl; when used alone, can produce outward calm with mental restlessness, so should be used with narcotic; can cause hypotension and extrapyramidal side effects; do not use in patients on antiparkinsonism therapy; not analgesic; potent antiemetic
Fentanyl and droperidol (Innovar)	Small titrated doses i.v.	Fixed combination of fentanyl and droperidol (each mL contains 0.05 mg fentanyl and 2.5 mg droperidol): after initial dose, usually best to use individual components to achieve specific effects required
Diazepam (Valium)	0.1 mg/kg i.v.	Benzodiazepine; useful for anterograde amnesia just before infiltration; irritation and/or phlebitis

[a] Although these drugs are the classic neuroleptanalgesic combination, they are often supplemented/modified by other narcotics or benzodiazepines (meperidine in 10–20 mg increments or diazepam in 1.25–2.5 mg increments).
Modified from Konovitch JW. Anesthetic management of the aging patient. In: Bosniak S, ed. *Advances in ophthalmic plastic and reconstructive surgery, vol II. The aging face.* Elmsford, NY: Pergamon Press, 1983;313; with permission.

ing barbiturate, such as methohexital (Brevital) 20 to 30 mg i.v. or thiamylal (Surital) 50 to 100 mg i.v., can be given conveniently just after the lids are demarcated but before they are infiltrated. This will obliterate any memory of the injections. Occasionally, several minutes of sneezing following the administration of methohexital will delay local infiltration. Midazolam (Versed) 1 to 2 mg i.v. may be administered alone or in combination with short-acting barbiturates just before local infiltration to accentuate antegrade amnesia. The combination provides the surgeon with a relaxed and easily arousable patient. Titrated doses of fentanyl (Sublimaze), droperidol, and fentanyl with droperidol (Innovar) can be used as needed (Tables 9A, 9B). Propofol (Diprivan) used as an infusion or in boluses is helpful during full-face laser resurfacing procedures. However, if frequent patient cooperation is desired during the procedure, no medication may be needed following lid infiltration.

It is exceptionally rare to find a patient who cannot be managed with the above techniques.

In general, the use of the CO_2 laser can significantly shorten the time required to perform the procedure and the amount of anesthesia needed.

Local Infiltration Anesthesia

Tetracaine 0.5% is applied topically to both corneas before the eyelids are scrubbed. Its onset of action is 20 seconds, and its duration is 9 to 24 minutes.

Opaque plastic corneoscleral protective lenses must be

TABLE 9B. *Newer neuroleptanalgesic agents*

Drug	Usual dose and route	Remarks
Midazolam (Versed)	1–2 mg increments i.v.	Painless injections, less local inflammation than diazepam; 3–4 times more potent than diazepam; pronounced anterograde amnesia, less anxiety and postoperative depression; can cause decrease in respiratory rate and tidal volume; no phlebitis
Methohexital (Brevital)	In small increments i.v.	Extremely short-acting; pain at injection site; respiratory depression; hiccups
Thiamylal (Surital)	In small increments i.v.	Same as methohexital
Ketamine (Ketalar)	i.v. or i.m.	Nonbarbiturate; "dissociative anesthesia"; used in titrated small doses, will not produce respiratory depression or hypotension; can be used with i.v. midazolam to prevent hallucinations
Propafol (Diprivan)	10 mg/mL gradual i.v. infusion or i.v. bolus	Sedative hypnotic agent, rapid onset and short sedation; i.v. infusion or intermittant i.v. bolus; patient's clinical response will determine infusion rate or frequency of incremental injection

applied to both eyes, promoting patient comfort and safety. When the CO_2 laser is used, polished nonreflective metallic corneal protectors must be used. Lidocaine 1% with 1:200,000 epinephrine will provide adequate lid anesthesia within minutes and will last approximately 90 minutes. Hemostatic vasoconstriction begins in about 5 to 10 minutes. The lids should be marked and injected before the surgeon scrubs to allow sufficient time for vasoconstriction before the initial incision is made. Diluting the epinephrine will minimize its cardiac irritation and possible dysrhythmia. Bupivacaine 0.25% to 0.75%, after a delayed onset of action, will anesthetize the lids for 4 to 12 hours. decreasing postoperative discomfort. A mixture of equal volumes of lidocaine 2% and bupivacaine 0.75% will provide a rapid onset of local anesthesia and prolong its duration.

Suture Materials

Various suture materials and techniques can be used in performing cosmetic blepharoplasty:

- *6-0 Black silk* is easy to handle and tie. It is soft, and the knots lie flat without difficulty. Although we have rarely seen this, some surgeons believe that if sutures are left in situ longer than 5 to 7 days, there is a tendency to form epithelialized suture tunnels. Others believe that these tunnels are formed by retained epithelial elements.
- *7-0 Black silk* has the same convenient intraoperative advantages as 6-0 silk, but with less tensile strength. It is easier to break when being tied and cannot be used for traction of the wound edge. The fine needle facilitates meticulous suture placement.
- *6-0 Nylon monofilament* suture material leaves minimal wound erythema and slides out of the wound easily on the fifth postoperative day, if placed in a continuous or subcuticular fashion. Intraoperatively, however, it is rigid and difficult to handle and tie.
- *6-0 Prolene* is soft, has no drag, is nonreactive, and is exceptionally strong. An initial double loop is essential to avoid knot slippage. 4-0 Prolene is used effectively for canthal tendon plication and has less of a tendency to produce granulomas.
- *Braided 6-0 nylon* handles as well as 6-0 black silk while causing less wound margin inflammation and erythema. Because of increased tissue drag, it is not as easy to remove as monofilament nylon.
- *6-0 Plain gut* is absorbable, does not require removal, and is virtually invisible. However, it is easily broken during the early postoperative period if there is marked swelling or if the lid is traumatized. On occasion, it may give rise to epithelialized suture tunnels and prolonged wound erythema. It is rigid, is difficult to handle and easy to break intraoperatively, and has considerable tissue drag.
- *6-0 Polygalactin* is ultimately absorbable but remains intact for at least 2 weeks. This handles well, approximating 6-0 black silk, but its use has none of the advantages of

6-0 plain gut and must be removed by the fifth postoperative day. If it is left in place until it absorbs, there may be prolonged wound erythema.

For medial and lateral canthal tendon plication or lid suspension, a variety of strong nonabsorbable sutures is available:

- *4-0 Mersilene* and *4-0 Polydek* are braided nylons that are easy to tie but have granulomagenic potential (Mersilene greater than Polydek).
- *Monofilament 4-0 Prolene* causes granulomas much less frequently but is difficult to handle, and the knots may slip.
- *Absorbable 5-0 PDS* is strong enough for canthal tendon suspension and is not absorbed for 2 months. It rarely causes granulomas, but because it is nonbraided, it can be difficult to handle, and the knots may slip.

Suture Techniques

Interrupted Sutures

Interrupted sutures may be used to perform primary closure or to supplement upper lid blepharoplasty closure utilizing running suture techniques. It will ensure accurate approximation of eyelid and direct browplasty wound margins. This suture technique is preferable for closure of upper lid incisions extending temporal to the lateral orbital rim and of upper lid laser incisions.

The suture must be passed at an equal depth on either side of the wound and must enter and exit at an equal distance from the wound edge (1 to 2 mm) to ensure accurate approximation of the wound edges. The suture must be tied just tight enough to appose the wound edges; excessive tightness may strangulate the wound margins. This technique permits the most exact approximation with the least trauma.

Running Locking Sutures

This technique has the advantage of a continuous suture tied only after the initial and final suture passages. Locking the suture after each bite avoids wound puckering. Suture removal is just as time-consuming as interrupted suture removal because each loop must be cut.

After the initial suture bite, the wound edges can be retracted with the suture, avoiding regrasping of the wound edge with forceps. As the needle is brought through the wound edge, it is grasped for placement of the next bite so that the needle will not have to be repositioned on the needle holder. The needle and suture are brought through a suture loop after exiting the wound edge, thereby locking the suture before placement of the next bite. Since there is a greater curvature of the superior wound edge, each bite of the superior wound edge must be placed slightly farther apart than the bite of the inferior wound edge. Some surgeons believe that this technique closes the wound too tightly and predisposes to prolonged edema.

Subcuticular Sutures

This is the preferred technique of many surgeons because the suture is easy to remove and does not leave epithelial suture tunnels. However, the wound often has to be reinforced with additional interrupted sutures. For this technique to be successful, accurate placement is essential. Monofilament nylon is an excellent material for this technique because of its ease of sliding through the tissue. The suture is placed several millimeters temporal to the wound edge, exiting in the lateral corner of the wound, first placed intradermally along the superior wound edge for 3 to 4 mm, then intradermally along 3 to 4 mm of the inferior wound edge. In a continuous fashion, the wound is closed with alternating intradermal placement along the superior and inferior wound edges. When the nasal end of the wound is reached, the suture is brought from the corner of the wound out through the skin several millimeters nasal to the wound edge. The free ends of the suture may be knotted on themselves, left loose, or fixated with a Steri-Strip. Sutures are removed on the fifth postoperative day. A 2-cm length of free suture may be left under a subcuticular in the middle of the lid. Traction on this suture will externalize the suture loop so that it can be cut, facilitating subcuticular suture removal.

Vertical Mattress Sutures

Vertical mattress sutures close the wound in two layers without leaving any buried suture material. This technique is effective in closing wounds in areas of tension and where wound edge eversion is desired. It is excellent for closing direct browplasty or midforehead wounds.

The suture is placed through the full-thickness skin flap inferiorly and superiorly 3 to 4 mm from the wound edge. It is then backhanded through the wound edge 1 mm on either side of the wound, closing the superficial dermis. The suture is tied inferior or superior to the wound.

Tissue Adhesives

Cyanoacrylate tissue glues can be utilized to close skin incisions. We have little experience with this technique. Conceptually, such glues will reduce the surgical time necessary for suture placement and eliminate the postoperative visit time by eliminating the need for suture removal. However, when upper lid myocutaneous resections and laser resurfacing are performed, greater control of the wound closure is necessary.

POSTOPERATIVE CARE

Cold compresses to the eyes must be applied in the immediate postoperative period and continue as frequently as possible during the next 72 hours. A multitude of devices can be used: iced-water washcloths, ice in a surgical glove, gel packs, frozen peas, computer-controlled cooling systems.

Erythromycin ophthalmic ointment is applied to the upper lid incisions and to uncovered resurfaced upper lids four times daily.

Laser and radiosurgery (Ellman International, Hewlett, NY) blepharoplasty techniques have significantly decreased postoperative discomfort, ecchymosis, and possibility of intraoperative and postoperative bleeding. Only mild analgesic medications are prescribed, usually acetaminophen, postoperatively. However, any complaints of severe, throbbing orbital pain should alert the surgeon to the possibility of retrobulbar hemorrhage. Sharp, stabbing ocular pain, usually with photophobia, denotes corneal desiccation and epithelial discontinuity. No patches are applied so that visual acuity can be monitored. Patients are informed that the application of ointment, as well as the tissue swelling, will cause blurring of vision, but any dimming of vision should not be ignored. Patients are instructed to call the surgeon immediately if that should occur. The application of iced compresses is continued at home, with patients keeping them in place for as long as they are comfortable, then removing them for 15 to 30 minutes before reapplying them. After 72 hours, they are discontinued. CO_2 laser blepharoplasty has markedly reduced postoperative swelling and the possibility of bleeding.

Laser facial rejuvenation patients will experience a different postoperative recovery. The areas covered with occlusive dressings may feel tight but not uncomfortable. The uncovered areas will feel hot, especially during the first 1 to 2 hours postoperatively. But this sensation will dissipate rapidly with frequent application of heavy emollients. If inadequately lubricated, the face will feel tight and uncomfortable. Usually, patients do not complain of pain, and in most cases there is very little discomfort. Discomfort not controlled with acetaminophen should alert the surgeon to the possibility of secondary bacterial or herpetic infection.

Sutures are usually removed between the fifth and seventh postoperative days. Earlier suture removal may decrease the formation of incision line suture cysts but increase the possibility of wound dehiscence. Lid margin sutures are left in place for 2 weeks. Mastisol and/or Steri-Strips may be applied to the wound if the sutures are removed before the fifth postoperative day.

CHAPTER 2

Skin: Anatomy and Physiology of Aging

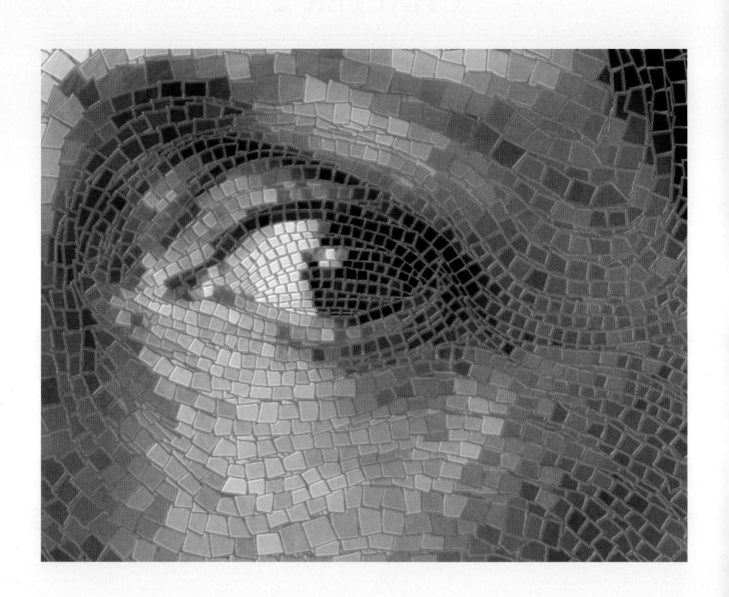

DEFINITIONS

Cutaneous aging is an dynamic process influenced by either intrinsic (chronologic) or extrinsic (environmental) factors. Intrinsic aging is manifested by the passage of time alone and is affected by genetics. Environmental aging is by far more responsible for aging skin; sunlight—ultraviolet (UV) light—is the main factor. Skin that manifests with chronic photoaging is recognized as photodamaged.

The following are the clinical abnormalities that characterize actinic-damaged skin:

- Dryness (roughness)
- Actinic keratosis
- Irregular pigmentation
- Elastosis
- Decrease in elasticity
- Increase in wrinkling

Histologically, these changes are represented by the following:

- Increased thickness of the stratum corneum
- Irregularity of the epidermis with occasional dermal inflammation
- Irregular dispersion of melanocytes
- Irregular aggregation of fibrous or amorphous material in the dermis
- Decreased glycosaminoglycans in the dermis
- Abnormal elastic fibers in the dermis

CLASSIFICATION OF SKIN TYPES AND LEVELS OF PHOTODAMAGE

Proper evaluation of the skin and its ability to tan or brown from UV exposure is very helpful in determining how patients will respond to laser treatment or chemical peeling, as well as predicting the surgical plan and prognosis regarding pigmentation abnormalities secondary to

TABLE 1. *Fitzpatrick's classification table*

Skin phototype	Skin color	Characteristics
I	White	Always burns, never tans
II	White	Always burns, tans minimally
III	White	Rarely burns, tans gradually and uniformly
IV	Light brown	Rarely burns, tans more than average
V	Brown	Rarely burns, tans profusely
VI	Dark brown or black	Never burns, deep tan

treatment. Fitzpatrick's classification table can be used for this procedure (Table 1):

- Skin types I to III, as a general rule, do not develop postinflammatory hyperpigmentation and are ideal candidates for laser resurfacing.
- Skin types IV to VI have a greater chance of developing postinflammatory hyperpigmentation or other pigmentary abnormalities.
- Skin types V and VI are often at risk for irregular hypopigmentation.

While Fitzpatrick's classification is very helpful in determining the risk of dyschromia associated with laser resurfacing, a classification is still needed that allows the surgeon to determine the type or level of photodamage and establish protocols for treatment of each patient.

A classification created by Dr. Richard Glogau may be helpful in trying to compare the efficacy of different treatments for certain skin types, although it still has its limitations, it tries to integrate different conditions, as well as use of makeup (Table 2).

Since there is no single ideal classification system that establishes the appropriate therapy, these are helpful when combined with the surgeon's clinical experience.

29

TABLE 2. *Glogau classification*

Damage	Description	Characteristics
Type 1 (mild)	No wrinkles	Early photoaging: mild pigmentary changes; no keratosis; minimal wrinkles Patient age 20s or 30s: minimal or no makeup; minimal acne scarring
Type 2 (moderate)	Wrinkles in motion	Early to moderate photoaging: early senile lentigines visible Patient age late 30s–40s: some foundation worn; mild acne scarring
Type 3 (advanced)	Wrinkles at rest	Advanced photoaging: obvious dyschromia; telangiectasis; visible keratosis; wrinkles visible at rest Patient age 50s or older: heavier foundation always worn; acne scarring that makeup does not cover
Type 4 (severe)	Only wrinkles	Severe photoaging: yellow-gray skin color; history of skin malignancies; wrinkles all over, no normal skin Patient age 60s or 70s: makeup cannot be worn (it cakes and racks); severe acne scarring

CHAPTER 3

Skin Therapies: Preparing the Patient for Surgery and Laser Resurfacing

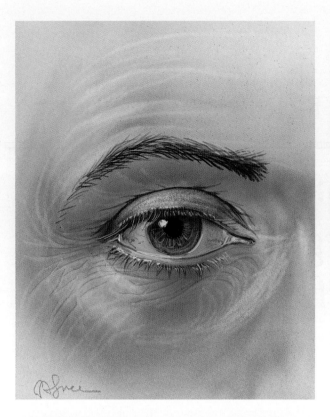

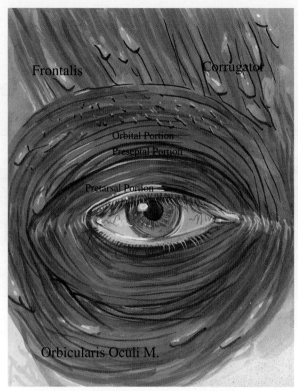

Frontalis

Corrugator

Orbital Portion

Presental Portion

Pretarsal Portion

Orbicularis Oculi M.

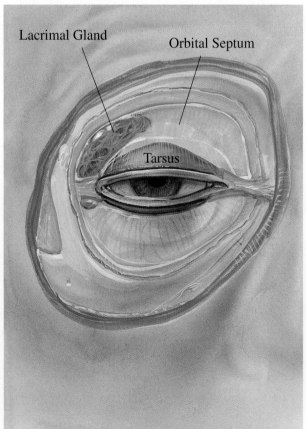

Lacrimal Gland

Orbital Septum

Tarsus

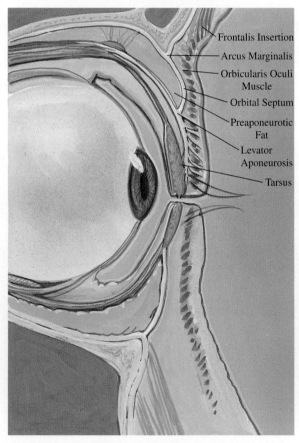

Frontalis Insertion

Arcus Marginalis

Orbicularis Oculi Muscle

Orbital Septum

Preaponeurotic Fat

Levator Aponeurosis

Tarsus

Skin care therapies, as well as the adequacy of a proper skin care regimen with its complexities, will maximize the results of cosmetic facial surgery and laser facial resurfacing. Skin care regimens are constantly evolving according to the season, climate, stress, general health, age of the patient, and pollution factors. They require a serious commitment by the patient to follow the instructions, which will include home care products and in-office therapies, such as cleansing facials, lymphatic drainage massage, and superficial peels (Fig. 1).

The aesthetician will be the liaison between the doctor and the patient and will be involved in improving the skin's appearance and readiness for the surgery. She will also provide psychologic help, reassurance, and comfort to the patient. The aesthetician should provide the following:

- Evaluation of the patient's skin: condition, level of hydration, level of elasticity, photodamage, ability to tan (see Fitzpatrick's classification; Chapter 2, Table 1), fluid retention, and periocular dyschromia.
- Evaluation of the patient's previous skin care regimen, with recommendations for adequate changes (e.g., proper

removal of face and eye makeup, explanation of benefits of regular skin care procedures that will maximize the results of surgery and protect patient's investment).

If the patient is not using any skin therapies, ideally, they should be initiated 2 or 4 weeks prior to surgery.

In general, the patient's skin care regimen would include the following:
Morning/night:

- Cleansing of skin
- Toning of skin
- Topical moisturizers enriched with antioxidants
- Retinoids (at physician's discretion)
- Alpha-hydroxy acids with or without bleaching agents (at physician's discretion)
- Sun block (only during the day and should be reapplied)

We also believe in nutritional supplementation and antioxidants. This is the right time to introduce or enhance these concepts in the patient's daily routine, since after their facial rejuvenation patients have an investment to protect and should be properly motivated.

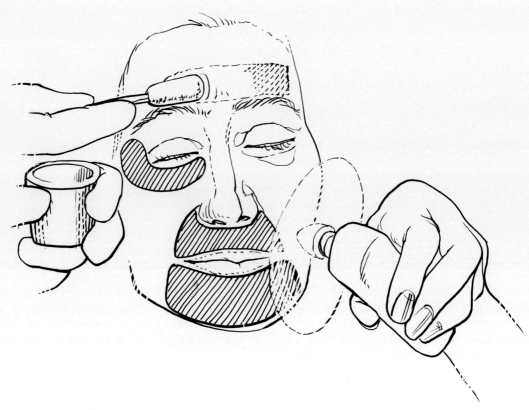

FIG. 1. After preparing the skin with home care products, in-office glycolic acid peels of varying strengths (30% buffered, 30% unbuffered, 50% buffered, 50% unbuffered, 70% buffered, 70% unbuffered) are used to improve skin texture and pigmentation and to prepare patients with thick, oily skin for laser resurfacing.

CHAPTER 4

Eyebrows: Anatomy and Surgical Techniques

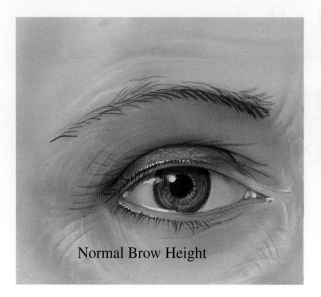

Normal Brow Height

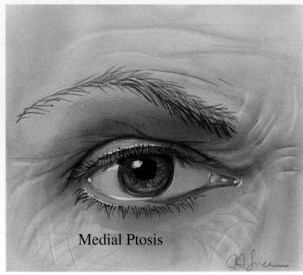

Medial Ptosis

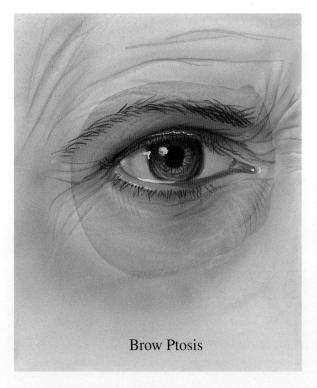

Brow Ptosis

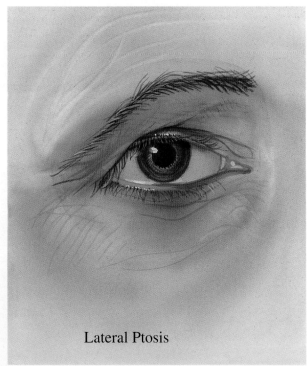

Lateral Ptosis

ANATOMY

The muscles innervated by the temporofrontal branch of the facial nerve—frontalis, corrugator, and procerus muscles—are responsible for upper facial and forehead expression and the resultant creases (Figs. 1, 2).

The thin, flat frontalis muscle, just deep to the forehead skin, extends from the galea aponeurotica at the vertex of the skull to the root of the nose and the eyebrows. Contraction of the frontalis creases the forehead and raises the eyebrows. The narrow bilateral procerus muscles extend from the superomedial orbital margin superiorly and laterally to the medial eyebrow. Their contraction lowers the eyebrow, pulls it nasally, and creates horizontal creases at the root of the rose. The narrow corrugator supercilii muscles are contiguous with the frontalis muscle in the midline, extending from the root of the nasal bones to the medial eyebrow. Their contraction creates vertical glabellar lines (Figs. 3A,B, 4A,B).

The superior orbital rim is a thickened portion of the frontal bone that serves to protect the globe. It sits anterior to the eyelids in a plane with the inferior orbital rim. The prominence and thickness of the superior orbital rim will affect the level and contour of the brow. A prominent, hyperostotic superior orbital rim with secondary anterior isplacement of the soft tissue of the brow will cast the superior sulcus and upper lid into deep shadow. Heavy, ptotic brows will cause secondary upper lid fold redundancy and/or temporal hooding.

The soft tissues overlying the superior orbital rim compose the eyebrow. There is a fat pad deep to the brow. Temporally, the eyebrow is attached to a bony ridge above the superior orbital rim. This support, weakened by aging, trauma, or facial palsy, may result in prominent temporal brow ptosis (Fig. 5). Although the density and contour of the brow follicles are altered by plucking, the idealized shape is tapered temporally, limited nasally at the medial end of the superior orbital rim and laterally at the junction of the superior and lateral orbital rims.

SURGICAL TECHNIQUES FOR BROW ELEVATION AND FIXATION

Our approaches to brow elevation, stabilization, and recontouring have changed dramatically since the last publication of this text. Our techniques have become less invasive and less traumatic, with higher patient acceptance and fewer potential complications.

Transblepharoplasty Internal Brow Suspension and Forehead Resurfacing

This is an effective, minimally invasive technique that can effectively stabilize ptotic brows and elevate them up to 2 mm. Preoperatively, with the patient in the upright position, the superior orbital rim is palpated, and the relationship between the brow and the superior orbital rim is noted; the number of millimeters of desired elevation is recorded. A marking pen denotes the nasal, central, and lateral brow segments that require elevation (Fig. 6).

An upper lid crease incision is made. A myocutaneous flap is elevated superiorly, exposing the suborbicularis fat overlaying the superior orbital rim (Fig. 7A). This fat is resected, exposing the periosteum of the superior orbital rim. The dissection begins laterally and ends medially, just lateral to the supraorbital neurovascular bundle (Fig. 7B). A series of 4-0 Prolene mattress sutures are anchored to the periosteum 4 mm above the superior orbital rim (Fig. 8A). They are attached to the orbicularis muscle just posterior to the eyebrow. The lid crease skin incision is closed. For additional support and eyebrow arch contouring, the forehead may be resurfaced using a carbon dioxide (CO_2) laser, with a band of laser applications extending from the brow to 2 cm above it (Fig. 8B). For more elevation, the entire forehead may be resurfaced.

Direct Brow Lift

As an alternate technique for higher brow elevation, direct brow resections can be used effectively (Fig. 9). This

(text continues on page 41)

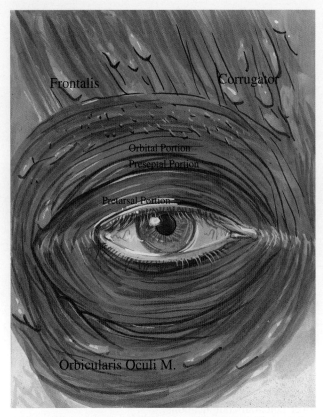

FIG. 1. The frontalis, corrugator, and procerus muscles are responsible for upper facial and forehead expression.

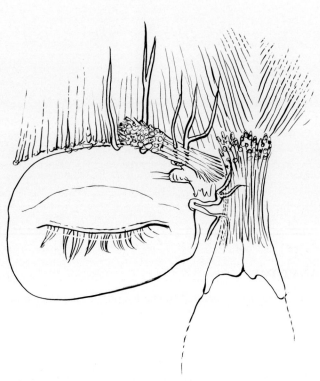

FIG. 2. The procerus muscles extend from the superomedial orbital rim to the medial eyebrow. Contraction of these muscles causes horizontal creases of the root of the nose. The corrugator supercilii extend from the root of the nasal bone to the medial eyebrow. Their contraction creates vertical glabellar lines.

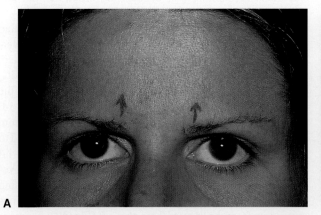
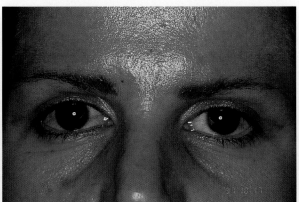

FIG. 3. A: This 34-year-old woman had prominent medial brow ptosis that caused a scowling appearance. **B:** Following transblepharoplasty internal brow suspension, lipocontouring of the brow fat pocket, lateral canthal suspension, and forehead resurfacing, her appearance is improved.

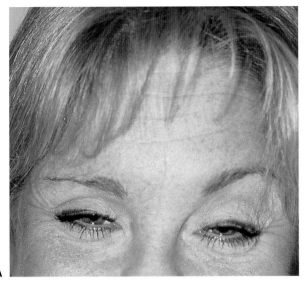 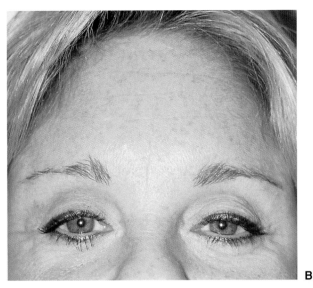

A   B

FIG. 4. A: Unconscious, habitual facial movements can cause characteristic facial asymmetries. This 37-year-old woman had chronic elevation of her left brow with transverse forehead rhytids. **B:** After Botox injections to the forehead and above the brow, her brow levels became symmetric and her forehead became smooth.

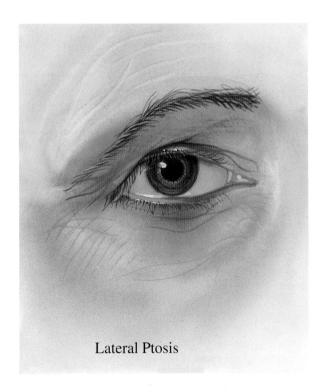

Lateral Ptosis

FIG. 5. Temporal brow ptosis is often the result of aging, tanning, or facial palsy.

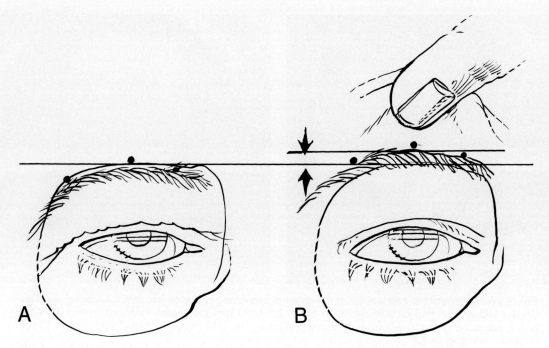

FIG. 6. The relationship between the ptotic brow and the superior orbital rim is determined. The required elevation is noted.

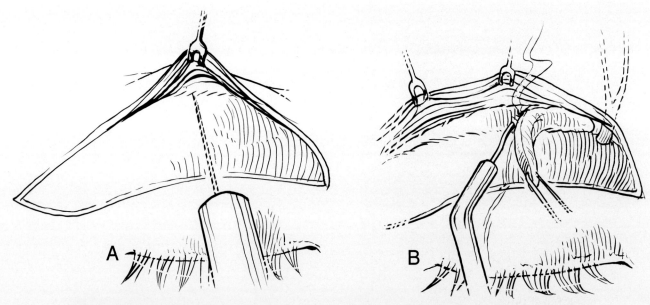

FIG. 7. A: A CO_2 laser or a radiosurgery electrode is used to develop the superior myocutaneous flap exposing the orbital rim. **B:** The suborbicularis muscle fat pad is resected as far nasally as the supra-orbital neurovascular bundle.

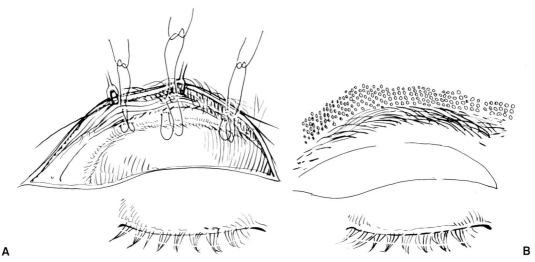

FIG. 8. A: 4-0 Prolene mattress sutures anchor the brow to the periosteum above the superior orbital rim. **B:** CO_2 laser resurfacing of the forehead supports the brow elevation.

can also be supplemented with CO_2 laser forehead resurfacing. This approach is particularly useful in cases of temporal brow ptosis with secondary dermatochalasis and temporal hooding of the upper lid.

This procedure is now reserved for patients with marked temporal hooding and lateral brow instability not adequately corrected with internal or endoscopic suspensions. The amount of elevation needed is determined preoperatively with the patient sitting in the upright position (Fig. 10) The surgeon can elevate the brow to the desired level by raising it with a finger or cotton-tipped applicator while a clear ruler with millimeter markings is placed over this area of measurement. The amount of elevation is determined in millimeters medially, centrally, and laterally. The brow contour can be tailored to the patient's desires and needs (Fig. 11). Direct brow temporal incisions are easily hidden and can be resurfaced with a CO_2 laser to make them even less visible (Figs. 12A,B, 13A,B).

This technique, however, is not effective for the correction of ptosis involving the medial portions of the brow. When such an incision is extended far medially, it becomes increasingly visible. When confined to the temporal portions of the brow, this technique is not only effective but also easily camouflaged. The most medial brow hairs are directed vertically. The brow hairs farther laterally are directed more laterally. The follicles at the superior margin of the brow are directed between 15 and 20 degrees downward; direct brow incisions should be angled downward at least 25 degrees to avoid transection of these follicles (Fig. 14). The direct brow incision technique necessitates meticulous closure, because the incision is in full view of the patient, as well as the surgeon (Fig. 15). There is no lid fold to be draped over the incision, as in upper lid blepharoplasty. The incision sits plainly on the brow but often is covered by long eyebrows. However, a superior migration of the incision, resulting in a visible scar, can occur if there is a postoperative loss of brow hair follicles.

There are instances when direct brow resection incisions can be placed in conveniently located deep forehead furrows (see Fig. 9). Even if these furrows are elevated in the midforehead, they can still be used effectively for incision

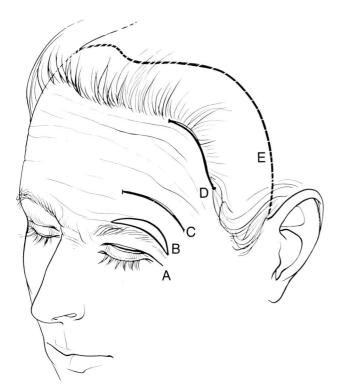

FIG. 9. The eyebrow may be elevated with resections placed **(A)** in the upper lid crease, **(B)** directly above the eyebrow, **(C)** in a midforehead crease, **(D)** at the hairline, or **(E)** in the scalp (bicoronal flap).

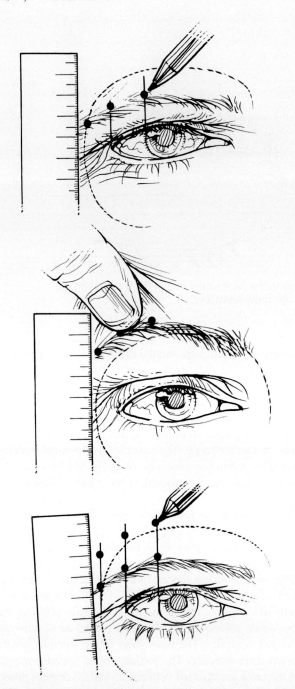

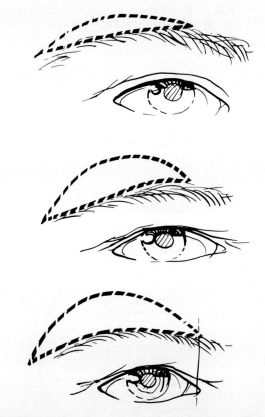

FIG. 10. Preoperatively, a clear ruler is used to determine the vertical height of the brow resection necessary to raise the brow to an appropriate level.

FIG. 11. Direct brow resections are tapered nasally and temporally and are never extended nasally beyond the medial canthal angle. These incisions can be resurfaced with the CO_2 laser at a later date.

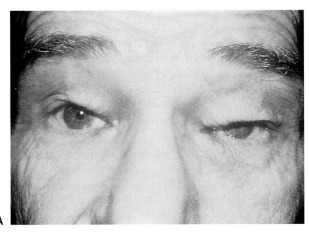
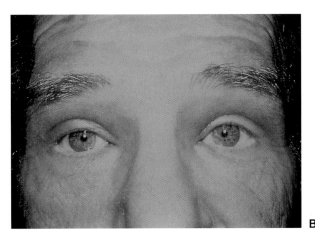

FIG. 12. A: This 45-year-old man had marked upper lid dermatochalasis secondary to recurrent inflammatory swelling of both upper lids. **B:** He has obvious improvement of his lid and brow levels and contours following upper lid myocutaneous resections, lipocontouring, levator aponeurotic repairs, direct brow resections, and CO_2 laser resurfacing.

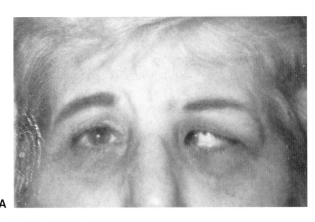

FIG. 13. A: This 59-year-old woman has prominent brow ptosis, upper lid redundancy, and strabismus. **B:** Following strabismus correction, upper lid blepharoplasty, lateral direct brow and medial midforehead resections, and glabellar Botox injections, she was significantly improved. **C:** Following full-face CO_2 laser resurfacing, she experienced further improvement and her forehead and brow surgical incisions were diminished.

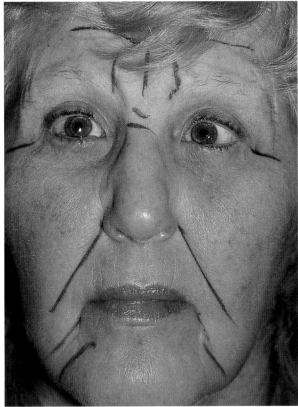
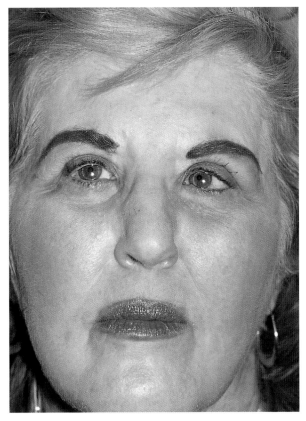

placement. Forehead furrow incisions are safer and more effective if higher furrows are used, avoiding frontal branches of the facial nerve. When using a forehead furrow, 50% more skin must be resected than if a direct brow resection is used. The midforehead technique provides an avenue for medial resections and can be used effectively to correct medial brow ptosis. CO_2 laser forehead resurfacing will augment all of the above procedures (see Fig. 13A–C).

In the modification of the brow contour, several factors must be considered. Temporal elevation leaving residual medial ptosis will create an unsightly scowl. The arch in women will be different from the arch and contour of the brows demarcated in men. In women, the most elevated portion of the brow arch should be at the junction of the middle two-thirds and temporal one-third of the brow, in line with the temporal limbus.

Brow elevation should not be excessively highly arched but should have a gentle upward sweep. The direct brow resection incision should be demarcated as tapering nasally and temporally but not extending any farther medially than the medial canthal angle (see Fig. 11). Nasal incisions in the brow often heal poorly and should not extend into the glabellar region. Temporally, they should not extend farther than the temporal-most extension of the brow and should not exceed the limits of the lateral orbital rim. These limitations can be modified if forehead furrows are being used to camouflage the incisions. The inferior incision should be placed just above the most superior cilia or within the uppermost two or three cilia. It should be remembered that if any of the hair follicles are transected by the incision, there will be a loss of eyebrow hair, and the incision placed directly within the eyebrow may be more exposed than intended postoperatively and may require secondary resurfacing.

After the incisions are demarcated, lidocaine 2% with 1:200,000 epinephrine is injected subcutaneously 10 to 15 minutes before the incisions are made. This can be done conveniently before the surgeon scrubs and before the patient is prepped and draped. The procedure can be performed bilaterally or unilaterally, in cases of unilateral brow ptosis secondary either to facial asymmetry, facial nerve palsy, or habitual facial posturing. A no. 15 Bard Parker blade, radiosurgical fine-wire electrode, or a 0.2-mm CO_2 laser handpiece is used to incise the previously demarcated incisions. The radiosurgical electrode (Ellman International, Hewlett, NY) should be used on the cutting mode, and the laser should be well focused to avoid lateral heat spread. When the inferior portion of the resection is incised, care should be taken to profoundly bevel (at least 25 degrees) the incising blade superiorly to avoid transecting the brow follicles (see Fig. 14). The superior portion of the resection is beveled in a complementary fashion to avoid a depressed scar. This facilitates wound closure, avoids depressed scarring of the brow, and promotes brow follicle growth through the superior wound edge. In completing the resection, additional care must be taken to ensure that the nasal and temporal edges of the resection form acute angles. This also will facilitate wound closure and the avoidance of dog ears at the nasal and temporal ends of the resection. The incision is made only through the thick brow skin. The underlying paper-thin frontalis muscle, galea aponeurotica, and periosteum should be left intact. The frontalis muscle protects the neurovascular arcades. It must be protected to avoid transecting the frontal branches of the facial nerve and the sensory branches. Deep nasal direct brow resections will affect forehead sensation and yield frontal anesthesia and hypoesthesia that may persist for up to 1 year postoperatively.

The wound may be closed in layers with absorbable su-

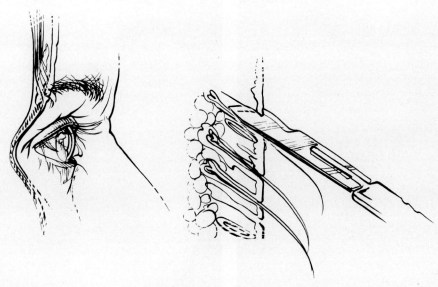

FIG. 14. A beveled incision avoids transection of the eyebrow follicles during brow resection and elevation.

ture used to close the undersurface of the skin. However, the use of removable vertical mattress sutures of 6-0 nylon not only gives adequate closure of the deep and superficial layers but also leaves no buried sutures as a nidus for granuloma formation. Brow resections in cases of paralytic brow ptosis and excessively unstable lateral brow position will require anchoring the brow to the underlying periosteum with nonabsorbable sutures to prolong the effect of the procedure; this effect can be furthered with CO_2 laser forehead resurfacing. The brow wounds must be closed in two layers—either with vertical mattress sutures or with a separate layer of buried nonabsorbable sutures (5-0 Prolene). A series of nylon sutures placed in a vertical mattress fashion is then used to meticulously close the wound, with care taken to evert the wound edges (see Fig. 15). Everting the wound edges decreases the likelihood of depressed brow scars. The wound is bisected with the first vertical mattress suture or buried suture, and each of the remaining halves of the wound is then bisected with the placement of the second and third sutures. The wound is continually bisected until apposition of the wound edges appears adequate. The superficial closure is then reinforced with a series of interrupted 6-0 nylon sutures. The nature of the brow skin and the location of the brow wound will necessitate more sutures than are required for closure of an upper lid blepharoplasty incision.

Men with thick brow skin or patients with a history of poor wound healing may be at risk for wound spreading. In these cases, the vertical mattress sutures should be left in place for 10 days, or buried 5-0 Prolene sutures should be used.

At the conclusion of the brow resection and repair, the upper lid folds and skin excess can be reevaluated. The lids are demarcated, and lidocaine 2% with 1:200,000 epinephrine is infiltrated subcutaneously. The upper lid demarcation and injection can be done after all the deep brow or vertical mattress sutures have been placed, but before the brow incision is closed completely, thereby determining the effect of the brow elevation and altered brow contour on the position and extent of the lid fold redundancy.

Bicoronal Brow Lift and Forehead Lift

Since the advent of internal suspension via transblepharoplasty or endoscopic approaches and the expanded use of botulinum toxin type A purified neurotoxin complex (Botox), the bicoronal technique of brow and forehead lifting has fewer indications. Patient acceptance of this technique has declined in the face of less invasive alternatives. It is indicated, and more accepted by patients, when other techniques have failed.

The bicoronal technique is not useful in bald patients or in those with high foreheads and receding hairlines who do not want their hairlines further elevated. The concept of a scalp flap folded in front of the face is alienating to most patients, who will decline to have this procedure performed. Some hair loss at the incision site (secondary to excessive tension on the incision) and damage to the supraorbital neurovascular bundle, with resultant frontal anesthesia or hypoesthesia and frontal nerve palsy, may occur.

During the night before surgery, patients are instructed to shampoo their hair for at least 10 minutes with an anti-

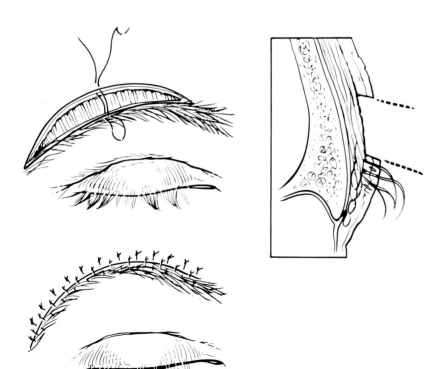

FIG. 15. Vertical mattress sutures of 6-0 nylon close the wound. Alternating interrupted sutures of the same material reinforce the skin closure.

bacterial solution. The hair anterior to the proposed incision is loosely braided or bound in sutures. A gullwing scalp incision is placed 8 cm posterior and parallel to the hairline, extending preauricularly just anterior to the superior helix of the ear, avoiding and protecting the lateral innervation to the scalp. Alternative approaches exist, including staggered hairline incisions that lower and redistribute the hairline, as well as foreshortening the forehead. The scalp can be shaved in a wide strip in the area of the proposed incision. However, this maneuver may be unnecessary or problematic.

Infiltration of lidocaine 1% with 1:200,000 epinephrine is used to establish a vascular tourniquet in this hypervascular area (Fig. 16A). The scalp incision site and proposed resection site are injected deeply along their full length, especially in the anterior portion of the flap. Inferiorly, the anesthetic hemostatic solution is infiltrated from the inferior extent of the scalp incision anteriorly to the lateral orbital rim, then superficially subcutaneously along the superior orbital rim, avoiding the large supraorbital vessels (and causing a glabellar hematoma), and across the root of the nose, along the contralateral superior orbital rim, laterally across the inferior aspect of the scalp incision, and again superiorly. This may be supplemented with a regional forehead block given with great care (supraorbital: inferior and posterior to the supraorbital notch and 10 mm along the orbital roof; supratrochlear: just inferior to the trochlea and 10 mm posterior to the rim).

The scalp and galea are incised preferably with a fine-wire radiosurgery electrode (blended cutting-hemostatic waveform) or a 0.2-mm CO_2 laser handpiece, leaving the pericranium intact (Fig. 16B). Laterally, the temporalis fascia is left intact. Lateral flap dissection must be kept deep to avoid branches of the facial nerve that run superficially at the superior orbital rim. Kocher clamps or Raney clips compress superficial bleeding of the wound edges. The anterior flap is elevated from the epicranium through the loosely adherent subgaleal plane: The gossamer fibers are easily lysed as far inferiorly as the superior orbital rim (Fig. 16C). Crosshatched CO_2 laser incisions of the undersurface of the anterior scalp flap allow easier retraction of the flap. The pericranium can be kept moist with sterile gauze that covers it and is stapled to the posterior flap. The superior orbital rim is exposed laterally. The procerus and corrugator muscles and the supraorbital and supratrochlear neurovascular bundles are carefully isolated. The procerus muscle is resected from the root of the nasal bone (Fig. 16D). This dissection is facilitated with the CO_2 laser or a fine-wire radiosurgery electrode. The supratrochlear nerve may be found within the superficial fibers of the corrugator muscle. Releasing this muscle from its bony insertion superiorly may avoid damage to the supratrochlear neurovascular bun-

dle before muscle resection. The palpated supraorbital notches may more easily aid in the location of the supraorbital neurovascular bundles, which are exceedingly variable and may have multiple rami and origins. The surgeon should trace the neurovascular arcades superiorly and avoid resecting the muscle–nerve junction.

The eyebrows are mobilized by releasing the galeal attachments to the flap. The subgaleal plane becomes less distinct as the superior orbital rims are approached, but the eyebrows cannot be elevated effectively unless they are released from the superior orbital rims. The areas of frontalis muscle incision are demarcated with 25-gauge needles placed through the skin–muscle flap at the nasal and temporal ends of forehead creases. Incisions 2 mm above and below each furrow will eliminate them. Since the nerves are superficial above the rim, resection at least 4 cm above the superior orbital rim minimizes the potential for sensory or motor nerve damage. The anterior skin–frontalis flap is retracted posteriorly and superiorly. The height of the flap resection will be determined by where it overlaps the superior wound edge and by the consequent eyebrow-elevating effect. The flap is elevated in the midline until the most caudal hairs of the medial eyebrows are 1 cm above the caudal-most supraorbital rim.

The scalp resection is usually between 1 and 3 cm in height (Fig. 16E). The amount of scalp resection must be twice as great as the amount of brow elevation desired. Care must be taken to ensure that the wound is not closed under excessive tension. A vertical incision of the flap, equaling the height of the proposed resection, is made in the midline. The edge of the resected flap is anchored with a 3-0 Dexon suture to the edge of the posterior flap. The flap is elevated 10 cm temporally until the lateral aspect of the eyebrow is raised 1 cm above the superior orbital rim, equaling the level of the medial aspect of the brow. The intervening galea is closed with 4-0 PDS sutures. The redundant anterior flap is incised perpendicularly where it overlaps the posterior flap and is anchored to the posterior flap with 3-0 nylon suture. The flap is elevated 4 cm from the midline, so that the point at the junction of the temporal one-third of the brow and the medial two-thirds of the brow is the highest point. The scalp is cut and anchored. The excess scalp between the anchoring sutures is excised, with care taken to bevel the resection and avoid transecting the follicles. The galea is closed with 4-0 PDS sutures.

The scalp is closed with medium-sized stainless steel staples, which are removed in 7 days (Fig. 16F). They are hemostatic and protect the hair follicles. A pressure dressing is not needed and may accentuate hair shock. A lightly applied, soft cling roll can be used as a dressing. Perioperative systemic antibiotics are preferred by some surgeons, as is topical antibiotic ointment.

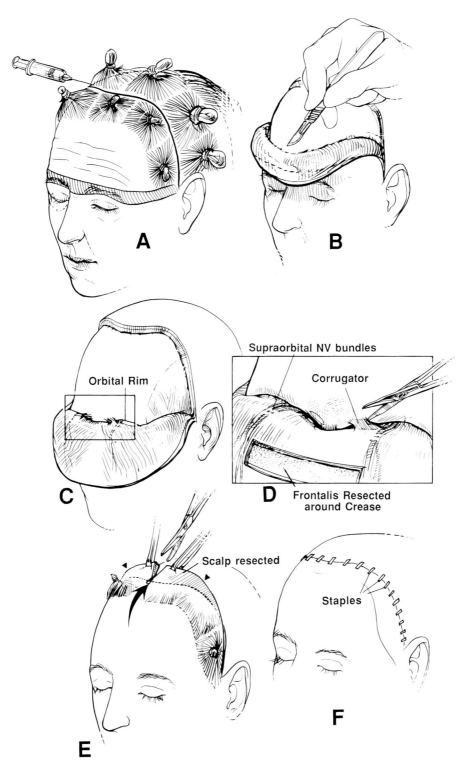

FIG. 16. A: The subcutaneous infiltration of lidocaine with epinephrine in the areas of proposed incision, undermining, and exposure establishes a vascular tourniquet. **B:** The loosely adherent gossamer fibers are dissected in the subgaleal plane. **C:** The superior orbital rim is exposed. **D:** The supraorbital and supratrochlear neurovascular bundles are exposed, as are the procerus and corrugator muscles. **E:** The anterior flap is incised vertically in the amount of the proposed resection. **F:** The wound is closed with stainless steel staples.

CHAPTER 5

Upper Lids: Anatomy and Surgical Techniques

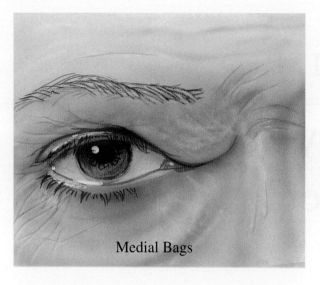

Medial Bags

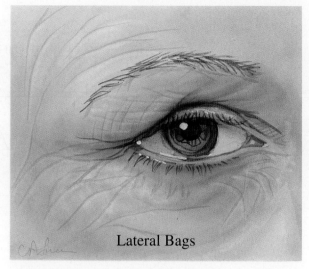

Lateral Bags

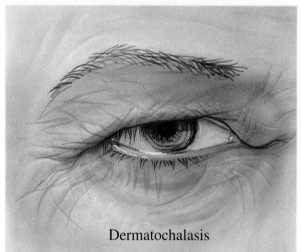

Dermatochalasis

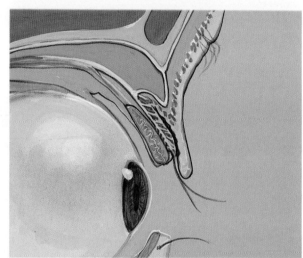

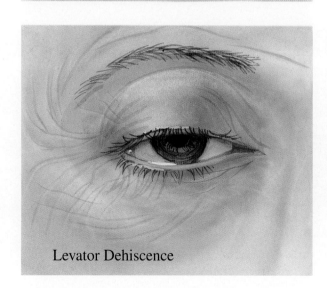

Levator Dehiscence

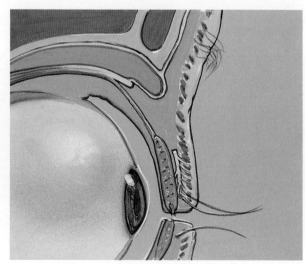

ANATOMY

The most conspicuous landmarks on the upper lid are the lid crease, lid fold, and superior sulcus.

Inferior to the brow, the superior sulcus of the upper eyelid is tucked under the superior orbital rim. In young, thin patients, the superior sulcus is a flat or concave surface. However, patients with prolapsed superior fat pockets have a shallower superior sulcus with a convex contour. The draped redundant skin in patients with severe upper lid dermatochalasis may completely obliterate the superior sulcus, creating a pseudoptosis obscuring the superior lid margin (Figs. 1A,B, 2). Elderly patients with orbital fat atrophy have hollow, deep superior sulci. The deep superior sulcus may be accentuated by levator aponeurotic disinsertions with lid crease retraction (Fig. 3).

The delicate multilayered structures of the upper eyelid are intimately related (Fig. 4). The lid crease, a critical surgical landmark, is formed by the anterior expansions of the levator aponeurosis, which insert into orbicularis muscle and skin generally 8 to 10 mm above the lid margin, just inferior to the superior tarsal border (Fig. 5A–D). The lid fold—preseptal skin and orbicularis muscle—is draped over the crease. The pretarsal skin and orbicularis inferior to the crease are lightly adherent to the tarsus, giving a smooth contour to the supraciliary portion of the upper lid. The lid crease and fold will be retracted and hidden in the superior sulcus if there is dehiscence of the levator aponeurosis from the anterior tarsal surface. Asian patients who have variations of the aponeurosis–septum complex may have a low lid crease, a double lid crease, or no lid crease.

The orbital septum, contiguous with a fibrous band beneath the superior orbital rim, the arcus marginalis, travels inferiorly and fuses with the levator aponeurosis 10 to 12 mm above the superior tarsal border. The fused septum and levator aponeurosis join the anterior tarsal surface at the junction of the inferior one-third and superior two-thirds of the tarsus. This septal–aponeurotic relationship has signif-

icance in cosmetic eyelid surgery. Septal dehiscences or true septal hernias may cause eyelid bulges that may be clinically undifferentiated from eyelid bulges secondary to orbital fat hypertrophy with anterior displacement of an intact septum. In either group, surgical correction necessitates opening the orbital septum above its union with the aponeurosis, allowing the fat to prolapse, and then resecting or vaporizing it.

The surgeon must be aware that posterior to these preaponeurotic fat pads are the levator aponeurosis and levator muscle. Aponeurosis repair is conveniently performed during blepharoplasty (Fig. 6A,B). Once exposed, the aponeurosis can be used for reconstruction of the lid crease. Involutional, postoperative, and posttraumatic dehiscences of the levator aponeurosis are manifested by ptosis, an elevated lid crease, and a retracted lid fold. Repair of the levator aponeurosis without resection of excess lid skin may correct the lid level and palpebral aperture asymmetry but produce a redundant lid fold that abuts the upper lid lashes. Patients who had smooth upper lid contours preoperatively may have prominent convexities and draping of the fold after reapproximation of a dehisced levator aponeurosis, if concomitant myocutaneous resections are not performed.

Ten to twelve millimeters above the superior tarsal border, the sympathetic muscle of Müller leaves the posterior surface of the levator aponeurosis. It inserts at the superior border of the tarsus. Normally not visible after an upper lid skin–muscle resection, Müller's muscle and its prominent vascular arcade above the superior tarsal border are well exposed if the levator aponeurosis is disinserted. If the surgeon is uncomfortable with repairing the levator aponeurosis during blepharoplasty, Müller's muscle provides an alternative route that can be used to correct 1 or 2 mm of ptosis from a conjunctival approach in conjunction with blepharoplasty.

Upper lid blepharoplasty incisions can be conveniently hidden in the lid crease. If an obvious lid crease is not visible or one exists at an undesirable level, an incision is demarcated between 8 and 12 mm above the superior lash

(text continues on page 54)

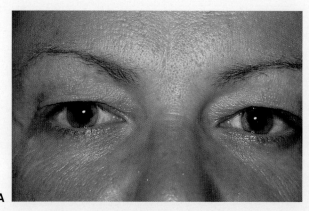
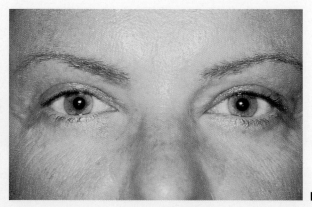

FIG. 1. A: This 40-year-old woman had marked upper lid fold redundancy obscuring her upper lid lashes. **B:** Following myocutaneous resections and lipocontouring, she has a well defined and natural upper lid crease.

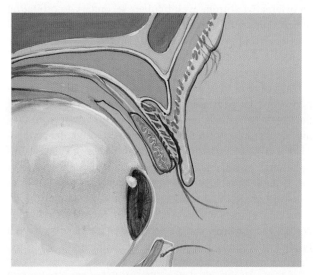

FIG. 2. A markedly redundant upper lid fold may obscure the upper lid margin and create a pseudoptosis.

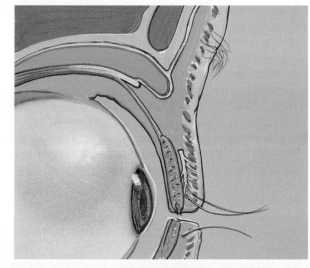

FIG. 3. Levator aponeurotic disinsertion will cause a retraction of the lid crease and accentuate a deep superior sulcus.

FIG. 4. Upper left: The upper lid crease is typically 8 to 12 mm above the lid margin. The lid fold is gently draped over the fold. The brow is at or slightly above the level of the superior orbital rim. **Upper right:** The frontalis, corrugator, supraciliaris, and procerus muscles support the brow and are responsible for its animation. The concentric pretarsal, preseptal, and orbital portions of the orbicularis muscle animate the eyelids. The pretarsal portion is tightly adherent to the overlying pretarsal skin. The preseptal skin is less adherent to the preseptal portion, forming the lid fold. **Lower left:** The orbital septum is fused with the levator aponeurosis 10 to 12 mm above the superior tarsal border. The levator aponeurosis inserts on the anterior tarsal surface and is adherent to the palpebral lobe of the lacrimal gland, which sits in the lacrimal fossa. The tarsal plate is approximately 34 mm in length and 10 to 12 mm in height. Upper lid fat pockets are most common nasally and centrally. **Lower right:** The orbital septum fuses with the levator aponeurosis before the levator inserts onto the tarsus. The preaponeurotic fat pad separates the septum from the aponeurosis above the level of septal–aponeurotic fusion.

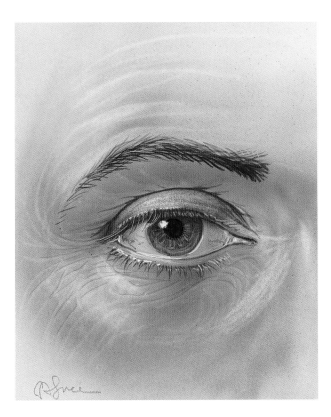

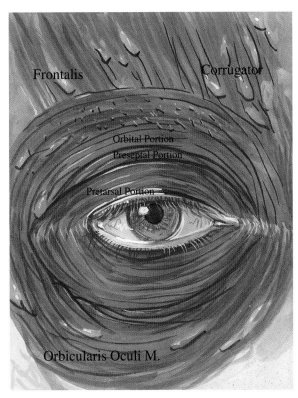

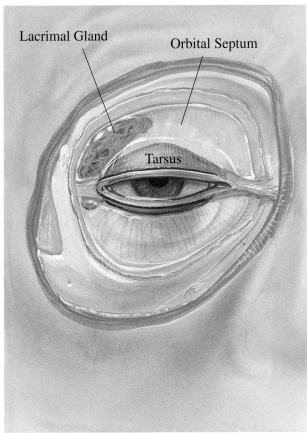

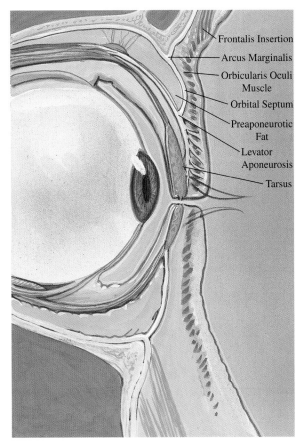

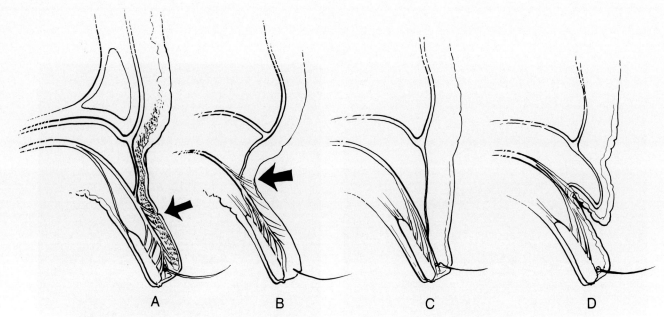

FIG. 5. The upper lid crease–fold complex: normal variants. The upper lid crease–fold complex is presumably formed by the anterior expansions of the levator aponeurosis. **A:** It is typically 8 to 10 mm above the lid margin. **B:** However, an elevated insertion may produce a high crease and deep superior sulcus that may give the appearance of a levator aponeurotic disinsertion. **C:** A weak or low anterior insertion of the aponeurosis will yield a low or inconspicuous lid crease. **D:** Redundant preseptal skin will accentuate the lid fold and may completely obliterate the lid crease.

line in non-Asian patients. A lid–fold complex nearer than 8 mm to the upper lid margin may create an appearance of skin redundancy and not yield a pleasingly flat contour to the upper lid and superior sulcus. Lowering an elevated lid crease may be accomplished easily; raising a depressed upper lid crease, however, is more difficult.

DRAPING THE PATIENT

The head drape should be placed firmly around the patient's head without raising or lowering the brow level or distorting the brow or lid crease contours. Lateral tension distorting the lateral canthus is also to be avoided. It is helpful to bring the body drape under the patient's chin and clamp it laterally to the head drape just anterior to the patient's ears, leaving the patient's face exposed and eliminating any feelings of claustrophobia that often arise while confined under the drapes. It also allows the patient's breathing to be monitored easily.

A plastic self-adhesive drape often makes the patient feel confined; in addition, it distorts the periocular anatomy, making lid level alignment and recontouring difficult. Plastic

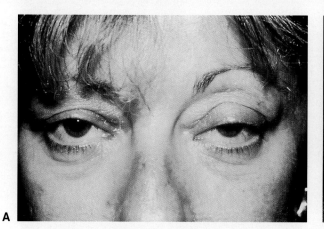
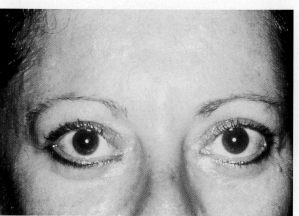

FIG. 6. A: This 36-year-old woman had upper lid crease asymmetry secondary to levator aponeurotic disinsertions. **B:** Following upper lid levator aponeurotic repairs, myocutaneous resections, and lipocontouring, as well as lower lid lipocontouring, retractor recessions, and lateral canthal suspensions, her appearance is improved.

self-adhesive drapes should be avoided or used only with great care. If the drapes pull superiorly, artificially elevating the brows, this will secondarily elevate the upper lid skin fold, making an inappropriately small resection seem adequate. The surgeon may not become aware of this until the drapes are removed and the patient sits up. Temporal distortions will affect the shape and contour of the lateral extensions of the upper lid resections. When using the carbon dioxide (CO_2) laser for making the incisions, the sterile drapes should be either moistened cloth (not paper) or sterilized heavy duty tinfoil.

EYE PROTECTION

During all facial rejuvenation procedures, the patient's eyes must be protected with corneal-scleral shields (opaque plastic when cold steel or radiosurgery (Ellman International, Hewlett, NY) is used; nonreflective metal when a CO_2 laser is used).

DEMARCATING THE UPPER LID INCISION

With the patient seated in an upright position, the superior aspect of the incision is demarcated, with care taken to keep 8 to 10 mm from the brow (Fig. 7). When the patient is supine but before the patient is prepared and draped, the upper lid crease incisions are demarcated (Fig. 8). The demarcation lines may be made with any dye that will not be removed completely when the patient is prepared. Toothpicks dipped into methylene blue or vital green or sterile gentian violet marking pens are useful for this purpose. A scalpel blade may be used to sharpen the blunt tip of a prepackaged marking pen. A cotton-tipped applicator moistened in alcohol can be used to remove extraneous or inaccurate markings. The inferior extent of the upper lid resection is marked with methylene blue at the level of the desired lid crease. There may be multiple existing creases from which to choose, but one should be selected at least 8 to 10 mm superior to the lashes centrally that gives a sufficiently elevated lid fold and a flattened contour above the lashes. In patients with a low lid crease, an appropriate level must be selected. The contralateral lid crease incision must be measured and reproduced exactly. Conversely, an existing elevated lid crease secondary to levator aponeurotic disinsertion is too high, and an appropriate incision should be made more inferiorly on the lid.

Nasally extending the incision beyond the superior punctum invites medial canthal webbing, unless a Burrow's tri-

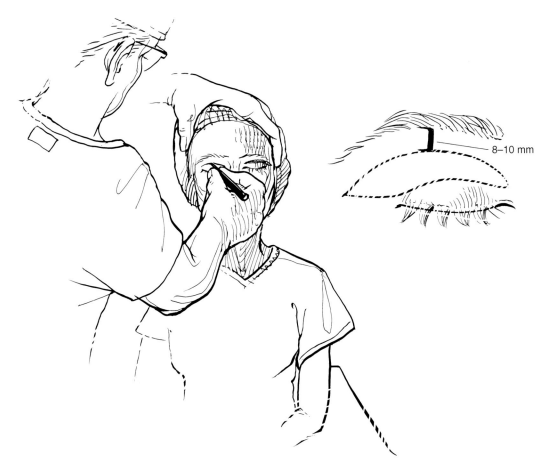

8–10 mm

FIG. 7. The superior aspect of the upper lid myocutaneous resection is demarcated with the patient in the upright position. Care is taken to maintain an appropriate distance from the brow.

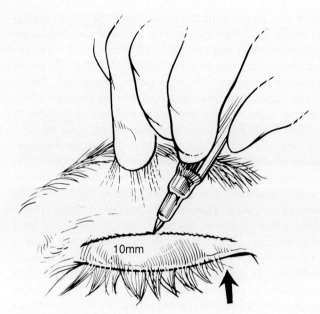

FIG. 8. The inferior extent of the upper lid resection is demarcated at the level of the desired lid crease.

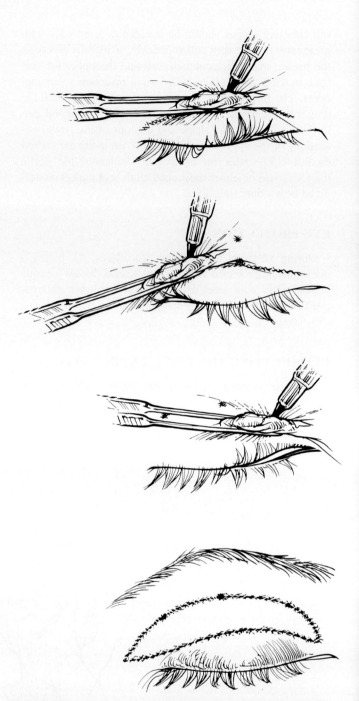

FIG. 9. Smooth Adson forceps grasp the redundant lid folds to ensure that too much skin has not been demarcated for resection.

angular flap is interpolated. The resting tension lines medial to the punctum are absolutely transverse. Since a hollowed medial sulcus may need at least as much skin to cover it as the preoperative convexity, aggressive skin resection is never appropriate in this location. Medial skin resection must be done with extreme caution. CO_2 laser resurfacing is often more effective than an extended medial resection in reducing medial redundancy.

The incision may be modestly continued temporal to the lateral orbital rim just above a smile crease, if there is residual slight temporal hooding. Since the incorporation of CO_2 laser resurfacing into eyelid rejuvenation, the myocutaneous resections must be even more conservative to allow for cutaneous tightening. If a CO_2 laser is used in the continuous-wave mode to incise the skin, the incisions should be made on the inside of the demarcation lines because of the small zone of lateral heat spread.

Significant temporal hooding requires correction of brow ptosis with a brow supportive procedure. This decision must be made preoperatively. The superior extent of the resection is first determined centrally after the brow level and contour have been established.

After demarcation, with the patient sitting, the superior extent of the desired resection is noted, with care taken to maintain an appropriate distance from the resection to the brow (see Fig. 7). Smooth Adson forceps grasp the redundant lid fold tangentially to ensure that too much resection has not been demarcated (Fig. 9). This must be done gently without forced eyelid closure. The amount of skin grasped should be marked conservatively. A distance of 8 to 10 mm between the upper margin of the resection and the brow should be left. The width of the grasp is widened, and the amount of tissue grasped is increased; the surgeon should

note when the upper lid lashes are mildly everted. The skin at the superior edge of the forceps is marked with methylene blue or gentian violet. The lid fold is grasped, and the excess is demarcated nasal and temporal to the central point. A curvilinear line joins these three points at the superior extent of the resection with the nasal and temporal ends of the inferior aspect of the resection. Care is taken to form tapered ends with acute angles at either end of the resection. The shape of this resection will vary from patient

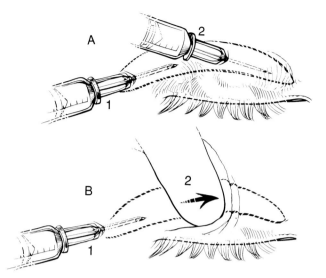

FIG. 10. A: The standard multiinjection technique with a 30-gauge needle to infiltrate the upper lid. **B:** To avoid ecchymosis secondary to subcutaneous infiltration, the local anesthetic is carefully injected temporally and then massaged nasally across the lid.

to patient, depending on the amount of lid fold redundancy, the contour of the brow and lid crease, the canthal angle, and the smile creases. The patient is asked to open and close the eyes to ensure proper selection of lid crease and adequate lid closure. When demarcation of the incisions is complete, the patient is comfortably sedated, and the lids are infiltrated subcutaneously using a short 30-gauge needle. Since there is usually no bleeding with upper lid CO_2 laser resections, it becomes critical to avoid provoking any hematomas during lid infiltration. To this end, injecting a subcutaneous wheal of anesthetic laterally and massaging it across the lid is an effective, minimally traumatic technique of infiltration (Fig. 10)

SKIN RESECTION

After opaque corneal protectors are placed on each cornea, the previously demarcated incisions are incised with a no. 15 Bard Parker blade, fine-wire radiosurgery electrode, or 0.2-mm CO_2 laser handpiece. To avoid incision irregularities, one smooth continuous stroke is used for the lower incision. The subcutaneous infiltration distends and immobilizes the tissue, facilitating the incision. Effective countertraction along the incision site facilitates this maneuver (Fig. 11). When a CO_2 laser or radiosurgery electrode is used to incise the skin, it is helpful to moisten the site first to minimize any possible charring. Seated to the side of the table, the surgeon can easily draw the blade,

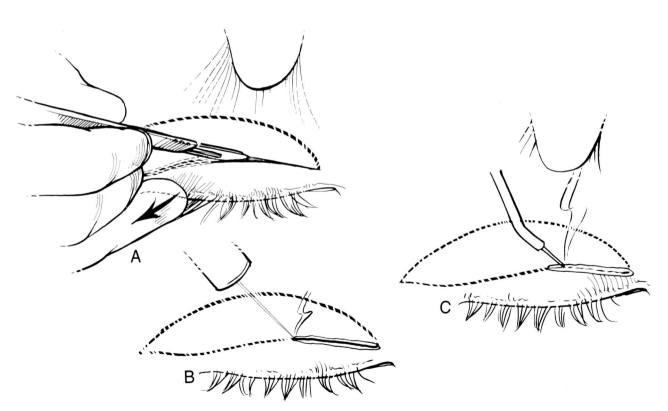

FIG. 11. With effective countertraction, the cutaneous upper lid incisions are made with a scalpel, CO_2 laser, or fine-wire radiosurgery electrode.

CO_2 laser handpiece, or radiosurgery electrode toward him-or herself, incising the wound nasally to temporally. Care must be taken to incise the previously demarcated incisions accurately, preserving the acute nasal and temporal angles of the resection. The temporal tip of the skin flap is lifted with a 0.5-mm forceps; anterior traction is applied. Wesscott scissors, a fine-wire radiosurgery electrode, or a 0.2-mm CO_2 laser handpiece is used to sharply dissect the posterior aspect of the skin flap at the anterior surface of the orbicularis muscle (Fig. 12). Blunt dissection is not appropriate, since no areolar plane exists. The hydrodynamics of subcutaneous infiltration of local anesthetic facilitates the dissection.

At the nasal end of the wound, care is again taken to preserve the acute angle of the skin flap. A medial or lateral Burrow's triangular resection or CO_2 laser resurfacing can be performed, if necessary, to reduce apparent skin excess medial or lateral to the resection. The resected skin should be placed in a moistened saline sponge until the wound has been closed. After wound closure, if CO_2 laser resurfacing is not to be performed, the surgeon may expect slight upper lid eversion if sufficient skin has been resected. Maintaining an appropriate distance between the brow and the superior edge of the resection is most critical and will reduce the risk of overresection. The subcutaneously injected an-esthetic will result in apparent lagophthalmos. If the lids can be closed passively, no skin has to be replaced in the upper lid. If the wound cannot be closed without severe lagophthalmos or marked ectropion, a segment of resected skin must be grafted into the appropriate position (50% overcorrection is necessary, since the graft will contract). Before regrafting is attempted, the head drape should be loosened to ensure that the lid margin deformity is real. The cautious surgeon can even save the resected skin in a Petri dish filled with saline and store it in a refrigerator until several days after surgery.

Skin resection alone has limited application. It can be used in cases of thin lids with adequate lid creases and excessive lid folds but without hypertrophic orbicularis muscle or fatty prolapse.

SKIN–MUSCLE RESECTION

The demarcation and incision of a skin–muscle flap is exactly the same as the demarcation and incision of a skin flap. However, the dissection differs. At the temporal tip of the wound, the skin and orbicularis muscle are grasped with a 0.5-mm toothed forceps; a fine-wire radiosurgery electrode, a 0.2-mm CO_2 laser handpiece, or Wesscott scissors is used to buttonhole the orbicularis. Continued anterior

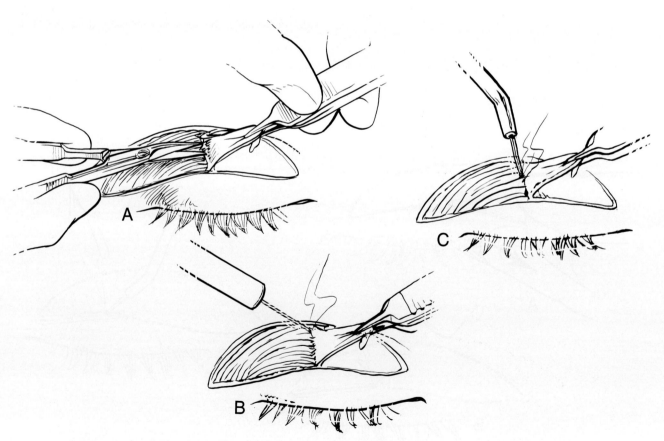

FIG. 12. Wesscott scissors **(A)**, a 0.2-mm CO_2 laser handpiece **(B)**, or a fine-wire radiosurgery electrode **(C)** is used to resect the skin flap.

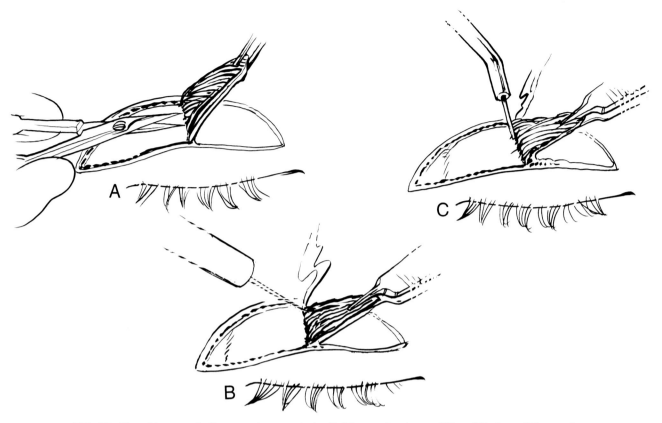

FIG. 13. The skin–muscle flap may be resected with Wesscott scissors **(A)**, a CO_2 laser **(B)**, or a fine-wire radiosurgery electrode **(C)**.

traction is applied to the skin–muscle flap with a toothed Adson forceps as the flap is dissected sharply off the anterior aspect of the septum. Deep incision will open the septum and yield fat prolapse, alerting the surgeon not to deepen the plane and injure the levator aponeurosis. As with a skin flap, attention to leaving acute angles at the nasal and temporal wound edges is critical for meticulous wound apposition (Fig. 13).

The skin–muscle flap provides easy access to the orbital septum and prolapsed orbital fat pockets. Resecting orbicularis muscle with skin will also better define the lid crease. A strip of orbicularis muscle may be resected separately at the level of the desired lid crease. However, we prefer to accentuate the crease by resecting a band of orbicularis the full width of the skin resection (Fig. 14A,B). This technique is most useful in patients with thick, boggy

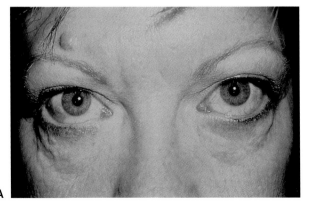
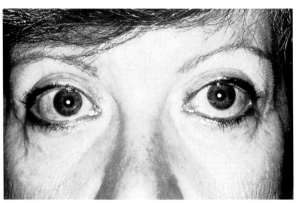

FIG. 14. A: This 54-year-old woman had thickened, boggy upper lids. **B:** Her upper lid contours improved with myocutaneous resections, lipocontouring, and suborbicularis brow fat resection.

lids, subcutaneous fatty deposits, and low set, flat, prominent brows, obscured superior sulci, and generously draped upper lid folds. When combined with brow suborbicularis fat resection, this technique not only defines the crease–fold complex but also sculpts the anterior lid contour and creates a visible superior sulcus. If the patient wishes to change the brow contour, brow elevation may also accentuate the deepened sulci and well defined lid creases.

RESECTING STEATOBLEPHARON

Adipose tissue within the lid is predominantly postseptal and preaponeurotic. Theoretically, there is also a postaponeurotic fat pad, but practically this is rarely of consequence. Septal weakness or rarefaction will allow anterior prolapse of the fat or a true herniation of the fat. Additionally, obese patients and Asian patients may have subcutaneous and preseptal fatty deposits. The latter ectopic fat is effectively removed with skin–muscle flap resection. Preaponeurotic fat may be handled using a variety of techniques (Table 1).

SEPTAL CONTRACTION

If there is little fatty prolapse when gentle pressure is applied to the globe, the preaponeurotic fat septum can be contracted and the superior sulcus recontoured with direct application of cautery, radiosurgery electrode touched to a forceps, or defocused CO_2 laser.

SEPTAL BUTTONHOLE

Gentle pressure on the globe will accentuate the convexities of incipient fatty prolapse. The septum is buttonholed with Wesscott scissors, a fine-wire radiosurgery electrode, or a 0.2-mm CO_2 laser handpiece at the most prominent point on the anterior bulge. The bright yellow fat of the temporal pockets or the whitish fat of the nasal pocket is prolapsed through small septal openings with continued pressure on the globe (Fig. 15). If scissors or scalpel is used, a curved hemostat is used to clamp the base of the fat flush with the septum. The fat is shaved off the anteriorly curved surface of the clamp. The anterior surface of the clamp is cauterized with a cautery or radiosurgery electrode. Care is taken to retract the skin and to avoid any contact of the conductive clamp with the skin. The base of the resected fat is grasped with a toothed Adson forceps before the clamp is released (Fig. 16A–E). If there is a bleeder, it can be localized and cauterized before retracting into the orbit.

OPEN-SKY FAT RESECTION

For complete visualization of the superior sulcus, the open-sky technique is utilized. The septum is buttonholed with Wesscott scissors, a fine-wire radiosurgery electrode,

TABLE 1. *Management of steatoblepharon*

Septal contraction
Cautery
Radiosurgery
CO_2 laser
Fat resection
Cold steel
Cautery
Radiosurgery
CO_2 laser
Direct CO_2 laser vaporization

or 0.2-mm CO_2 laser handpiece and then opened to the full width of the skin incision or resected if it is thick and adds bulk to the lid. This maneuver also provides enhanced visualization of the fat pockets. Gentle pressure on the globe accentuates fat prolapse. The prolapsed fat is resected. Cautery or a defocused CO_2 laser is used when a large vessel is identified in a fat pocket (Fig. 17A–E). When radiosurgery is employed, the vessel is grasped with a fine forceps, and the electrode touches the forceps (cutting, hemostatic, or blended waveforms can be used with equal effectiveness). The nasal fat pocket is often more vascular, requiring cautery applied to large vessels that are visualized as the fat is resected. Bipolar cautery (Fig. 18) or radiosurgery, as well as a defocused CO_2 laser handpiece, can be used to shrink the prolapsing fat.

MEDIAL BULGE

Correcting upper lid medial bulge may be problematic. It may be the manifestation of a prolapsed medial fat pocket, draping of excessive medial canthal skin, or apparent dermatochalasis secondary to medial brow ptosis. Resecting skin in that area requires astute observation and precise judgment. Little skin need be resected if a medial fat pocket is removed, since the resultant concave sulcus contour requires as much skin as the preoperative convex contour. In addition, subcutaneous contraction follows fat pad resection, particularly when the CO_2 laser is used to vaporize the fat.

However, the greatest difficulty arises if a medial brow ptosis is unrecognized. Skin resection will merely accentuate the medial bulge and the brow ptosis. A brow elevation must precede eyelid resection for effective correction. However, a brow elevation procedure performed after aggressive skin resection will result in severe lid lag and lagophthalmos.

SKIN RESECTIONS NASAL TO THE SUPERIOR PUNCTUM

Extending a crescent-shaped skin resection nasal to the superior punctum can cause vertical shortening of the an-

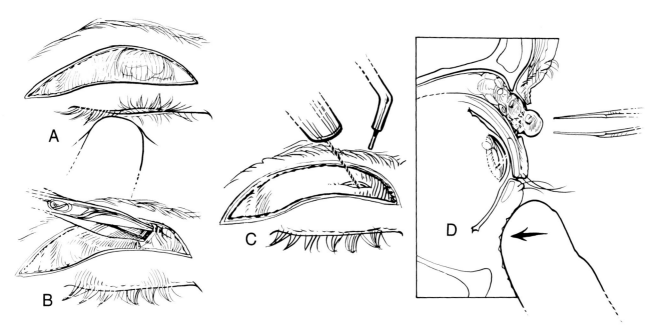

FIG. 15. **A:** Gentle pressure on the globe accentuates fatty prolapse. The septum can be opened with Wesscott scissors **(B)**, a fine-wire radiosurgical electrode **(C)**, or a CO_2 laser. **D:** Opening the septum anterior to the advancing fatty convexity will allow the fat to be expressed through the septal buttonhole.

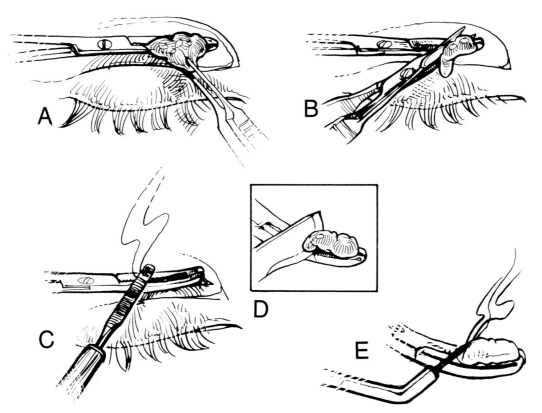

FIG. 16. **A:** The fat is stabilized with a curved hemostat and **(B,D)** shaved flush with the clamp. **C:** The base of the clamp is cauterized. Care must be taken to avoid contact of the clamp and the skin. The base of the fat pocket is grasped with toothed Adson forceps before the clamp is released. Any bleeders can be identified before the fat is allowed to retract into the orbit. **E:** A fine-wire radiosurgery electrode can be used to shave and coagulate the fat simultaneously.

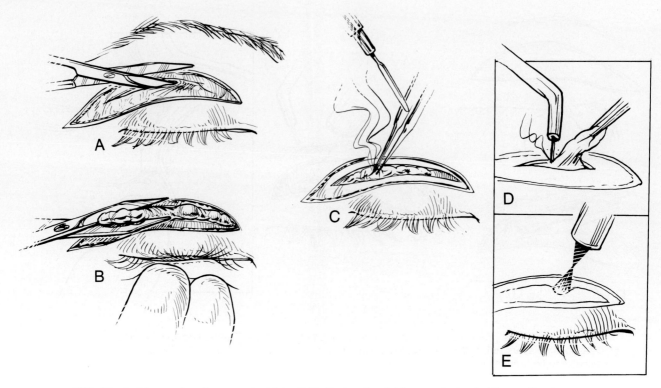

FIG. 17. A: The septum is opened widely. **B,D:** Prolapsing fat is resected with Wesscott scissors or a fine-wire radiosurgery electrode. **C:** When blood vessels are identified, they are grasped with a forceps and touched with a radiosurgery electrode. **E:** They may also be ablated with a defocused CO_2 laser.

terior lamella of the lid medially, without effectively removing the medial bulge. Techniques that increase the area of the skin resection without shortening it vertically are useful here. CO_2 laser resurfacing will reduce medial overlap without extending the lid crease incision.

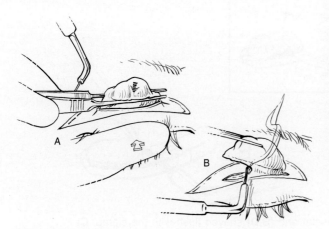

FIG. 18. If a CO_2 laser is not used once the septum is opened, a bipolar forceps can be used to grasp the prolapsing fat and shrink it. The pedicle of prolapsing fat can be resected without bleeding using a fine-wire radiosurgery electrode (using a blended waveform).

Burrow's Triangle

Several millimeters lateral to the extreme nasal and superior extent of the resection (the exact distance and length are determined by the location of the medial bulge), an incision is made perpendicular to the superior edge of the resection. Adjacent tissue is undermined, and the skin flaps are overlapped.

The width of the base of the triangular resection is determined by the amount of overlap necessary to reduce the medial skin excess without causing excess traction nasally on the side of the nose or the medial aspect of the superior sulcus, and without distorting the medial canthal angle or superior punctum. The overlapping area is trimmed in a triangular fashion, the base contiguous with the primary resection and the apex directed medially and superiorly. The defect is closed with interrupted sutures.

Medial W-plasty

The superior and inferior aspects of the upper lid skin resection are extended as far nasally as necessary to encompass the medial bulge (more medial than the superior punctum). The two incisions are joined in a W-plasty rather than directly with a curvilinear incision. This provides two triangular areas of medial resection with minimal vertical traction. From the superomedial incision, an incision is demarcated at a 60-degree angle directed inferiorly and laterally. From the inferomedial incision, an incision is demarcated at 60 degrees, directed superiorly and laterally. The two angled incisions will intersect at a point. No undermining is indicated in this area, since this maneuver may lead to scar contracture and wound depression.

Laser Resurfacing

This is our procedure of choice in the management of cutaneous redundancy nasal to the superior punctum. After medial brow stabilization and medial lipocontouring, any residual medial skin redundancy can be addressed with laser resurfacing of the preseptal skin, extending as far nasally as necessary.

EXTENDING THE TEMPORAL RESECTION

If the upper lid skin excess is confined exclusively to the lid, there is no indication to extend the resection farther temporally, and it may be tapered acutely medial to the lateral orbital rim. Mild residual temporal hooding not corrected by temporal brow elevation, or an excessive fold overlying the lateral palpebral raphe may be addressed with modest lateral extension of the upper lid resection beyond the lateral orbital rim. If the temporal hooding is great, brow elevation, forehead or full-face CO_2 laser resurfacing, or rhytidectomy is indicated. The inferior edge of this resection should be at least 4 mm superior to the lateral palpebral raphe to avoid disturbance of the periorbital lymphatics, inadvertent contiguity with the lower lid incision, and rounding or distortion of the sharp lateral canthal angle. The shape of the temporal resection will be determined by the contour of the tissue to be resected. The inferior edge may follow a smile crease or resting tension line horizontally or may be angled slightly superiorly. This incision is easily blended into the lid crease incision, as long as it is not extended more than several millimeters beyond the lateral orbital rim.

LID CREASE FORMATION
AND WOUND CLOSURE

Resection of orbicularis muscle in addition to preseptal skin accentuates the formation of the upper lid crease. However, in patients with thick, boggy lids, additional maneuvers may be necessary. Welding the severed ends of the orbicularis muscle with cautery will increase subcutaneous fibrosis and deepen the lid crease (Fig. 19). CO_2 laser contraction of the pretarsal and preseptal orbicularis muscle will also create further definition of the lid crease–fold complex where necessary. Suture techniques can also be used. If the patient has a low lid crease, anchoring the inferior skin edge to the inferior edge of the levator aponeurosis will raise the crease and also make it more prominent. Three or four interrupted sutures will form the crease. Wound closure then can be completed with 6-0 black silk

or 6-0 nylon sutures, placed in a continuous, locking, interrupted, or subcuticular fashion. If a subcuticular suture is used, 6-0 nylon in preferable. A suture stent should be placed under a suture loop in the midline of the wound so that if there is any difficulty removing the suture, the stent can be elevated and the suture can be cut in the midline, facilitating its removal. We prefer to use interrupted 6-0 black silk sutures in patients who have had CO_2 laser incisions and eyelid skin resurfacing.

MANAGEMENT OF CONCOMITANT TRUE PTOSIS

In cases of extreme dematochalasis, a markedly redundant lid fold may obscure the superior lid margin and narrow the vertical palpebral aperture, creating a pseudoptosis. To measure the true vertical palpebral aperture (upper lid margin to lower lid margin), this fold must first be retracted. Conversely, redundant upper lid skin does not in and of itself narrow the vertical palpebral aperture. However, dermatochalasis is often associated with true blepharoptosis. If not recognized preoperatively or if the surgeon assumes that the narrowed vertical palpebral aperture is secondary to excessive lid soft tissue, there will be postoperative asymmetry of the palpebral apertures. In addition, for third-party reimbursement, it is important to document the constriction of the superior peripheral visual fields secondary to both pseudoblepharoptosis and true blepharoptosis. Ptosis secondary to large levator aponeurotic disinsertions with markedly elevated lid creases and septal retraction into the superior sulcus may mask the redundancy of the lid fold. After the levator aponeurosis has been approximated to the tarsus, the lid fold excess and fat pad prolapse may become apparent.

EXTERNAL LEVATOR APONEUROTIC REPAIR FOR CORRECTION OF APONEUROTIC DISINSERTION AND MODERATE PTOSIS

The upper lid blepharoplasty incisions are demarcated. Only enough local anesthesia is given for dissection and repair of the levator aponeurosis, avoiding akinesia of the levator. One-half milliliter of lidocaine 1% with 1:200,000 epinephrine is injected subcutaneously in the area of the previously demarcated lid crease incision. One-tenth milliliter of the same solution is injected subcutaneously in the midline of the upper lid just superior to the cilia. This allows the painless placement of a 4-0 silk lid traction suture in the gray line, if desired. The traction suture is clamped to the sterile drapes inferiorly, stabilizing the upper lid and keeping it at maximum stretch. The lid crease incision is made with a no. 15 Bard Parker blade, Wesscott scissors, a fine-wire radiosurgery electrode, or a 0.2-mm CO_2 laser handpiece. A skin flap is developed inferiorly to the level of the lash follicles. While the skin flap is retracted with small rakes, a 5-mm strip of pretarsal orbicularis muscle is resected, exposing the anterior surface of the tarsus (Fig. 20). Superiorly, blunt and sharp dissection develops a skin–muscle flap, exposing the anterior surface of the orbital

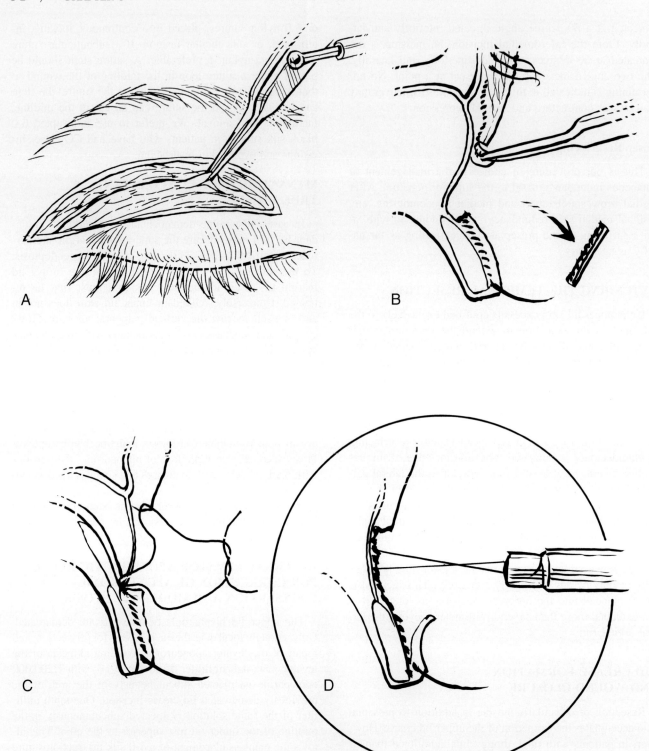

FIG. 19. The upper lid crease can be accentuated by welding the resected edges of orbicularis muscle, anchoring sutures to the levator aponeurosis, or contracting orbicularis muscle and septum with a defocused CO_2 laser.

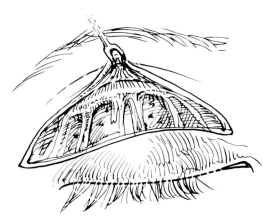

FIG. 20. While the skin flap is retracted anteriorly, an 8-mm strip of pretarsal orbicularis muscle is resected. This maneuver exposes the anterior surface of the tarsus, provides a surface for aponeurotic fixation, and precludes thickening of the lid after aponeurotic repair and advancement.

septum. If the levator aponeurosis is dehisced, Müller's muscle will be visible at the superior tarsal border. It can be identified readily by the prominent vascular arcade just superior to the upper margin of the tarsus. The shiny white inferior edge of the levator aponeurosis may be visible several millimeters above Müller's muscle. However, if it has retracted superiorly, it may not be visible until the septum is opened and the prolapsing orbital fat is retracted. The position of the aponeurosis can be confirmed by having the patient look up and down, watching the aponeurosis move, grasping the inferior edge, and feeling the pull on upward gaze. The orbital septum can sometimes be confused with the levator aponeurosis. Gentle pressure on the globe should cause the preaponeurotic fat to bulge and distort the septum. As the septum is fused with the levator aponeurosis inferiorly, there may be some movement with upward and downward gaze. When the septum is grasped and pulled inferiorly, its adhesion to the arcus marginalis at the superior orbital rim is easily palpated. Once the septum is opened, the preaponeurotic fat should be clearly visible. The levator aponeurosis has no adhesions to the arcus mar-

ginalis and is deep to the preaponeurotic fat pads. When the aponeurosis is grasped and pulled inferiorly, it cannot be palpated in the superior sulcus.

Three mattress sutures of 6-0 black silk are placed into the anterior tarsus at the junction of its superior one-third and inferior two-thirds. The lid is everted to confirm that the suture has not inadvertently been passed through full-thickness tarsus. The lid traction suture is released. Each arm of the mattress suture is passed through the levator aponeurosis 1 to 2 mm superior to its inferior edge (Fig. 21). One throw of each mattress suture is tied over a bolster of 4-0 silk. This bolster can be used to release the 6-0 silk mattress suture and facilitate adjusting the lid level and contour. The patient is asked to look up and down. After the lid level and contour are adjusted, the silk bolster is slid out from under the mattress suture, and the knot is completed with additional throws of the suture. If lid lag is evident, a suture inadvertently may have been passed through the orbital septum, or an aponeurotic–septal adhesion persists. In either case, the suture must be removed; all adhesions to the orbital septum must be lysed before the suture is replaced. Additional infiltration of the lid with lidocaine 1% and 1:200,000 epinephrine is then performed. The skin–muscle and fat resections are performed. The wound is closed, and the lid crease is created with a series of interrupted 6-0 black silk sutures, apposing the wound edges and taking a bite of the inferior edge of the levator aponeurosis (Fig. 22).

FASANELLA SERVAT PROCEDURE: CORRECTION OF MINIMAL PTOSIS

Although levator aponeurotic surgery is our procedure of choice, preoperatively, if two drops of oxymetazoline 2.5% applied to the superior palpebral conjunctiva raise the upper lid to the desired level, an alternate effective technique can be used—tarsoconjunctivomüllerectomy with Müller's muscle advancement (Fasanella Servat procedure). The skin–muscle blepharoplasty incisions are demarcated. Topical tetracaine 0.1% is applied to both corneas. One milliliter of lidocaine 2% with 1:200,000 epinephrine is injected just inferior to the supraorbital notch and 10 mm posterior

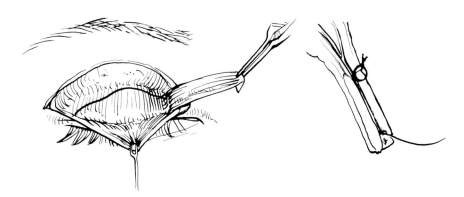

FIG. 21. The lid crease is formed, including the advanced inferior edge of the levator aponeurosis in the wound closure.

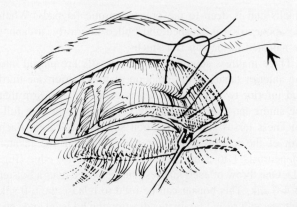

FIG. 22. 6-0 Black silk mattress sutures fixate the disinserted inferior edge of the levator aponeurosis to the anterior tarsal surface.

to the superior orbital rim. This supraorbital regional nerve block should anesthetize the middle two-thirds of the upper lid. The regional block is supplemented with subcutaneous infiltration of the same anesthetic solution along the lid crease and subconjunctival infiltration above the superior tarsal border. An opaque corneal protector is inserted.

The skin–muscle resection is completed. The lid is everted over a Desmarres retractor or curved hemostat (Fig. 23A). The superior margin of the tarsus is grasped with toothed Adson forceps and pulled superiorly, thus separating Müller's muscle from the levator aponeurosis. A curved hemostat with its concave surface facing inferiorly is clamped over the nasal one-half of the tarsus 4 mm above its everted superior border. Included in the clamp are 4 mm of tarsus, 8 mm of conjunctiva, and 4 mm of Müller's muscle (Fig. 23B). If there was an excessive response to oxymetazoline, the amount of tissue resected is decreased by 1 to 2 mm. If there was a suboptimal response, an additional 1 to 2 mm of Müller's muscle is resected. A second curved hemostat is similarly placed over the temporal one-half of the tarsus. Care is taken not to form a peak at the

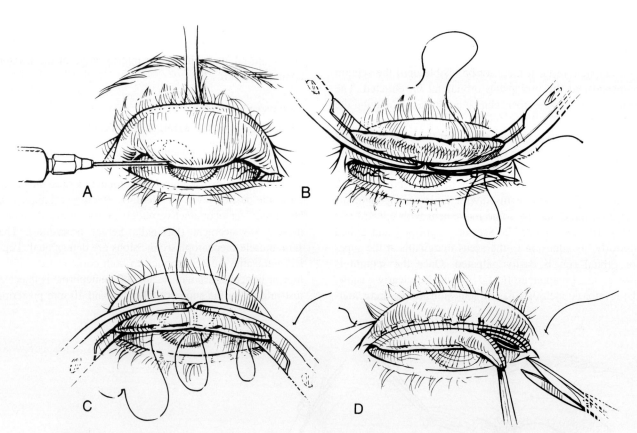

FIG. 23. A: The upper lid is everted over a Desmarres retractor. **B:** Curved hemostats, concave surfaces facing inferiorly, are applied 4 mm above the superior tarsal border. Included in the clamps are conjunctiva, tarsus, and Müller's muscle. A 5-0 monofilament suture is passed from the lid crease through full-thickness lid, exiting above the clamps through the palpebral conjunctiva. **C:** A running mattress suture is placed distal to the clamps, with each entrance bite placed immediately adjacent to the previous exit bite, leaving little exposed suture; it is angled at 45 degrees to facilitate suture removal. **D:** The tissue distal to the crush marks is resected.

junction of the two clamps. A 5-0 nylon suture on a C-2 needle is passed from the skin at the nasal extent of the lid crease through full-thickness lid, exiting through the nasal tarsus and palpebral conjunctiva just inferior to the clamp. The suturing is continued distal to the clamps in a running mattress fashion until the temporal end of the tarsus is reached. Each entrance bite is placed immediately adjacent to the previous exit bite (to minimize any exposed suture loops), angled at 45 degrees (to facilitate suture removal), and as close to the hemostat as possible (to avoid postoperative lid retraction) (Fig. 23C). The final suture bite is placed from the palpebral conjunctiva distal to the clamps through full-thickness lid, exiting in the skin in the temporal lid crease. The nasal clamp is released while the temporal lid is stabilized with the temporal clamp. The nasal tissue that was distal to the clamp is resected in the clamp marks (Fig. 23D). Care is taken not to cut the suture loops. The temporal superior tarsal border is grasped with a toothed Adson forceps. The temporal hemostat is released. The temporal tarsus, conjunctiva, and Müller's muscle are resected in the crush marks. The lid is inverted, and the posterior lamella is smoothed with a pass of the handle of the Adson forceps. The nasal and temporal ends of the 5-0 nylon suture are pulled medially and laterally to confirm that they will slide out without difficulty. They are then tied loosely to each other in the lid crease after the blepharoplasty wound is closed. Tying the Fasanella sutures too tightly will cause central peaking of the superior lid margin.

OTHER UPPER LID CONTOUR ABNORMALITIES

Not all smooth, dome-shaped upper lid convexities are prolapsed orbital fat. Gentle pressure on the globe exaggerating the prominence of the masses in their characteristic locations is the hallmark of prolapsed fat. Common chalazia are well circumscribed, firm, usually associated with inflammatory signs of the skin or palpebral conjunctiva, and located over the tarsus. Frontoethmoidal mucoceles often occur as dome-shaped masses in the medial superior sulcus, which in some instances can look like a medial fat pocket. However, they are firm, usually noncompressible, and contiguous with the orbital rims medially and superiorly. Dermoid or epidermoid cysts of the zygomaticofrontal or nasofrontal sutures, particularly those that have ruptured and are surrounded by an inflammatory pseudocapsule, may appear as an ill-defined temporal or nasal upper lid fullness or as discrete masses, mimicking a temporal or nasal fat pocket. These also, however, tend to be firm and noncompressible and may or may not be palpably adherent to the orbital rim. Tumors of the orbital lobe of the lacrimal gland may appear as temporal lid masses. They may be firm, noncompressible, adherent to the orbital rim, and associated with ptosis or proptosis.

Of most direct relevance to cosmetic blepharoplasty is the ptotic palpebral lobe of the lacrimal gland. It appears as a soft, compressible, movable mass in the temporal portion of the upper lid, where a distinct temporal fat pocket does not exist. It can be rolled between the examiner's fingers, and it may be unilateral or bilateral. On lid eversion, it is visible as a whitish gray mass at the superior temporal tarsal border. Prolapsed, ptotic lacrimal glands may occur with associated sarcoidosis, may be associated with obesity, rapid weight gain, recurrent lid edema, a hyperactive thyroid state, or Sjoïgen's disease, or may be a normal anatomic variation associated with shallow orbits, often seen in African-American patients.

The lacrimal secretory output usually is normal, and the condition is benign. For an acceptable cosmetic result after blepharoplasty in these patients, a resuspension or CO_2 laser contraction of the lacrimal gland is indicated.

RESUSPENSION OF THE LACRIMAL GLAND

Following demarcation of an upper lid skin–muscle resection, a skin–muscle flap is developed, exposing the orbital septum. The septum is opened. The palpebral lobe of the lacrimal gland is exposed just nasal to the lateral orbital rim, anterior to the lacrimal gland fossa. The periosteum of the lacrimal gland fossa is exposed with blunt dissection. Each arm of a double-armed, nonabsorbable suture (4-0 Polydek, 4-0 Prolene, or 4-0 Mersilene) is placed into the anterior surface of the ptotic lacrimal gland. Each arm of

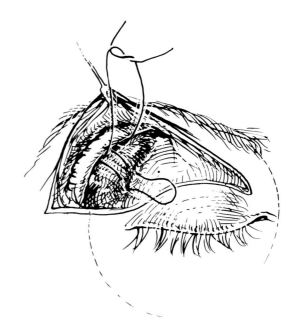

FIG. 24. A ptotic lacrimal gland can be resuspended to the periosteum of the lacrimal fossa with a nonabsorbable mattress suture.

the lacrimal gland suture is then placed through the periosteum of the lacrimal gland fossa behind the orbital rim (Fig. 24). If this maneuver does not adequately resuspend the gland, retracting it into the fossa, two holes can be drilled posterior to the superior temporal orbital rim, and the sutures can be pulled through them and tied. An alternative is CO_2 laser contraction of the palpebral lobe of the lacrimal gland. After exposure of the gland, its anterior surface is resurfaced with the CPG (computer pattern generator), causing a flattening of its anterior contour. This maneuver can be supplemented with suture suspension. The blepharoplasty wound is then closed.

CHAPTER 6

Lower Lids: Anatomy and Surgical Techniques

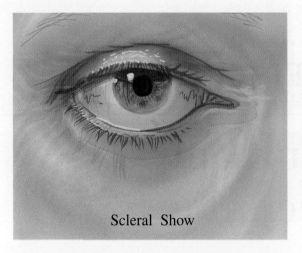

Scleral Show

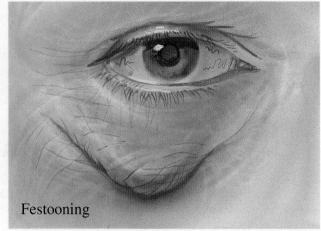

Festooning

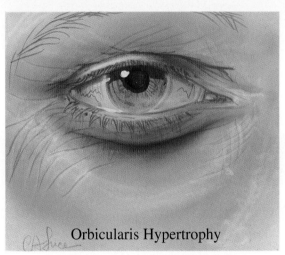

Orbicularis Hypertrophy

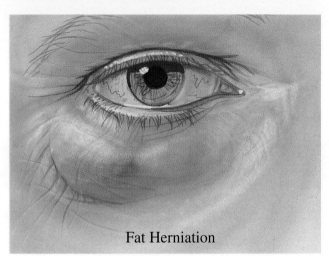

Fat Herniation

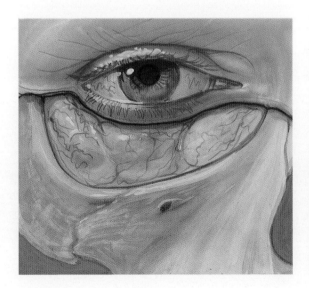

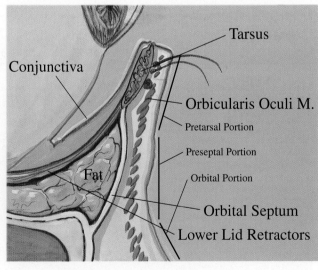

Conjunctiva

Tarsus

Orbicularis Oculi M.

Pretarsal Portion

Preseptal Portion

Orbital Portion

Fat

Orbital Septum

Lower Lid Retractors

ANATOMY

The relationship and relative levels of the medial and lateral canthal tendons may be racially predetermined and are certainly subject to congenital variation. In general, the lateral canthal angle is more acute than the media canthal angle. There is a prominently sharp angle at the outer canthus. Any rounding or distortion of this angle is quite visible. Congenital canthal tendon dehiscences or involutional canthal tendon laxity will alter canthal angle contours and potentiate any distortions of the horizontal palpebral fissure caused by lid surgery.

The lower lid structures are analogous to those of the upper lid but not as well defined (Fig. 1). The vertical height of the inferior tarsus is 4 to 5 mm. There is a lower lid crease, but it does not have the depth, prominence, or cosmetic significance of the upper lid crease, nor can it be

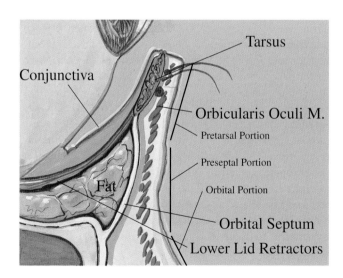

FIG. 1. Lower lid contouring can not be performed effectively unless the surgeon is intimately familiar with the complex interrelationship of the lower lid anatomic layers.

as effectively used to camouflage lid incisions. Meibomian glands are embedded within the tarsal plate, with orifices in the lid margin posterior to the lashes and anterior to the gray line. These cutaneous landmarks now have less surgical importance as transcutaneous lower lid incisions are rarely indicated.

The lower lid level and contour have several normal variations that must be considered before lid surgery is contemplated. The idealized lower lid rests at the level of the inferior limbus (Fig. 2A–C). Patients with high myopia, shallow orbits, proptosis, and thyroid lid retraction may have asymmetric or symmetric inferior scleral show (Fig. 3). Before the advent of the transconjunctival approach, cosmetic lower lid surgery in such patients had to be approached cautiously. Skin incisions alone and skin or skin–muscle resections accentuated inferior scleral show. Lateral canthal support remains essential when skin resurfacing is planned. If there is inadequate lateral canthal support, rounded, blunted lateral angles can result.

The inferior lacrimal excretory system is dependent on normally functioning lower lid structures and is very vulnerable during and after transcutaneous lower lid cosmetic surgery. Contraction and relaxation of the pretarsal orbicularis muscle, preseptal orbicularis muscle, and the superficial and deep tendons of each of these muscles contribute to the lacrimal pump mechanism, assisting the flow of tears into the puncta and through the canaliculi, lacrimal sac, and bony nasolacrimal duct. Involutional stretching of the canthal tendons and orbicularis muscles will not only alter the lower lid levels and contour but also distort the horizontal palpebral aperture and decrease the effectiveness of the lacrimal pump. The result is a functional and cosmetic deformity characterized by a deep, static tear lake and symptomatic epiphora (tears running down the cheek). The act of wiping away the tears aggravates the lower lid laxity. The transconjunctival approach to the lower lid leaves the lacrimal pump undisturbed and can be combined with lateral canthal plication, when necessary.

71

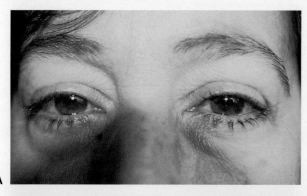

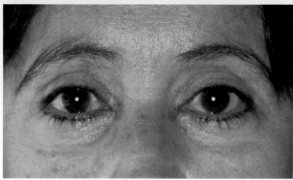

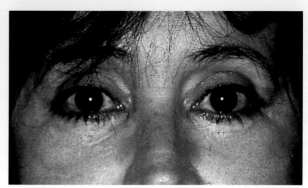

FIG. 2. A: This 50-year-old woman had moderate lower lid fatty prolapse and moderate upper lid heaviness with mild to moderate rhytidosis. **B:** Her lid contours are improved following lower lid transconjunctival lipocontouring, upper lid sculpting, and levator aponeurotic repairs. **C:** Her lid contours were further improved following laser resurfacing.

The normal punctum is completely hidden by the eyelid and sits in tight apposition to the globe. If the punctum is visible without touching the lower eyelid, it is considered everted. Everted puncta are not in the most efficient position for tear drainage. Furthermore, puncta exposed by chronic medial ectropion may become dry and obliterated by complete keratinization. Gravitational effects and the heavy lower facial musculature make any lower lid skin or skin–muscle subciliary incisions risky. Transcutaneous lower lid incisions hugging the cilia also risk canalicular disruption if they are carried nasal to the punctum.

Familial or acquired septal weakness or dehiscence with prolapse or incipient prolapse of orbital fat is responsible for secondary lid surface convexities. These convexities may be accentuated by excessive subcutaneous fatty deposits, edema (most often secondary to cardiovascular dysfunction, renal insufficiency, chronic allergic dermatitis, or intermittent cutaneous edema of unknown etiology), or hyperactive thyroid–induced orbital infiltration. Malar hypoplasia may accentuate fat pockets, creating a gutter between the inferior orbital rim and the prolapsed fat pockets. Prominent diffuse lower lid bagginess will completely obliterate the fat pad contours and may be secondary to hypothyroid myxedema, senescence, or actinic elastotic degeneration with decreased skin turgor and resilience (Fig. 4). This redundancy may accentuate the lower lid crease, create excess folds along resting tension lines and drooping over the inferior orbital rim, or festooning over the malar eminence. Hypertrophic pretarsal orbicularis muscles, particularly prominent in younger patients with animated facial expression and not related to involutional changes, may create a horizontal ridge across the lower lid (Fig. 5); these may be asymmetric and are accentuated by having the patient smile.

Involutional laxity of the canthal tendons has a marked effect on the level and contour of the lower lid margin. Gravitational effects on atonic lids accelerate these changes, causing extreme laxity or dehiscence of the canthal tendons

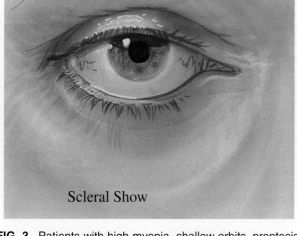

Scleral Show

FIG. 3. Patients with high myopia, shallow orbits, proptosis, or thyroid disease may have inferior scleral show. Inferior scleral show may also be a normal variant.

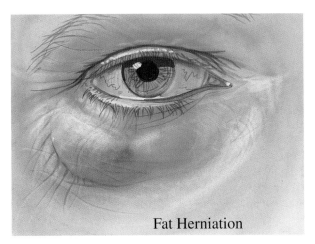

Fat Herniation

FIG. 4. Diffuse fatty prolapse of the lower lids may obliterate the individual fat pad contours.

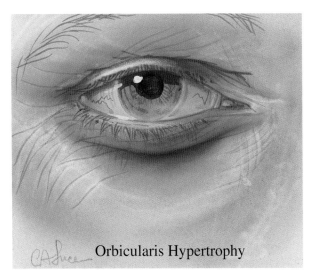

Orbicularis Hypertrophy

FIG. 5. Lower lid hypertrophic orbicularis muscle creates a horizontal ridge across the lower lid.

in patients with facial palsy. Epiphora secondary to a weakened lacrimal pump mechanism may contribute to medial canthal tendon laxity, because patients are constantly wiping tears away from their flaccid eyelids. Epiphora may be further accentuated by medial ectropion with punctal keratinization and by aberrant regeneration with gustatory lacrimation.

DRAPING THE PATIENT

Passing the body drape under the patient's chin and clamping it to the head drape laterally eliminate any distortion of the lower lids and facilitate the assessment of intraoperative lower lid laxity. Plastic adhesive drapes may distort the lateral canthi and lower lid margins. Drapes pulling the lower lids inferiorly may lead to lateral canthal distortions.

GENERAL SURGICAL PRINCIPLES

The patient is comfortably sedated preoperatively. Intraoperatively, an intravenous short-acting agent is given before infiltration of the lids. The patient then will be arousable later during the procedure and immediately afterward.

If only lower lid transconjunctival lipocontouring is to be performed, subconjunctival infiltration (Fig. 6B) is supplemented with an infraorbital regional block or an inferolateral peribulbar block (Fig. 6A). A mixture of equal amounts of lidocaine 2% and bupivacaine 0.45% with 1:000,000 epinephrine and sodium bicarbonate 0.1% in each 10 mL of anesthetic is used for infiltration.

If laser resurfacing is to be performed at the same time as blepharoplasty, the entire length and height of the lids are infiltrated laterally from the lateral palpebral raphe, temporal to the orbital rim, as far nasally as the inferior punctum, from just beneath the lashes superiorly to the level of the orbital rim inferiorly. Medial canthal tendon surgery

will require subcutaneous infiltration extending more nasally, anterior to the anterior lacrimal crest on the lateral wall of the nose.

In our opinion, the transcutaneous approach to lower lid blepharoplasty is obsolete. A skin or skin–muscle flap is not necessary for exposure of the lower lid fat pockets, and skin resection is only necessary on rare occasions when there is an extreme excess of lower lid skin.

Redraping of the lower lid skin after transconjunctival lipocontouring often does not require additional incisions of the lower lid skin. Residual lower lid rhytidosis can be reduced with resurfacing using a carbon dioxide (CO_2) laser and/or an erbium:yttrium-aluminum-garnet (Er:YAG) laser (Fig. 7A–C). In patients with extreme excess, a pinch technique can be used to perform a conservative skin resection, with the incision camouflaged in the lower lid crease. This is best performed 3 months following lower lid laser resurfacing.

The lower crease is demarcated. The redundant skin is grasped with a fine-toothed forceps, its vertical excess demarcated. If grasping this amount of skin does not deform the lid margin, it can be resected (Fig. 8A,B). The resection is tapered nasally and temporally. The wound is closed with interrupted or running sutures.

TRANSCONJUNCTIVAL LOWER LID BLEPHAROPLASTY

After topical anesthetic is applied to the cornea, a protective corneal-scleral lens is inserted [opaque plastic for cold steel and radiosurgery (Ellman International, Hewlett, NY), nonreflective metal for laser use].

The lower lid margin in everted with a small rake, Desmarres retractor, or a 4-0 black silk traction suture. The

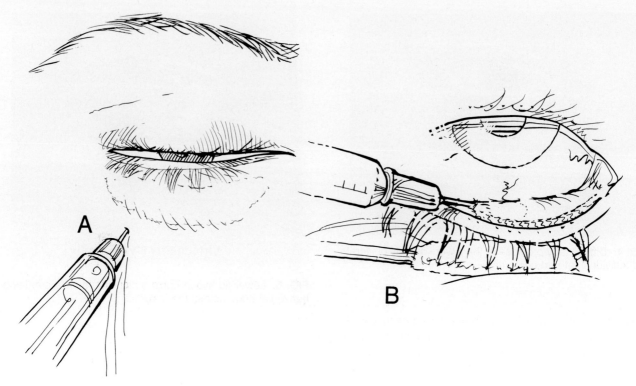

FIG. 6. A,B: An inferior peribulbar block supplements subconjunctival infiltration when a transconjunctival blepharoplasty is performed.

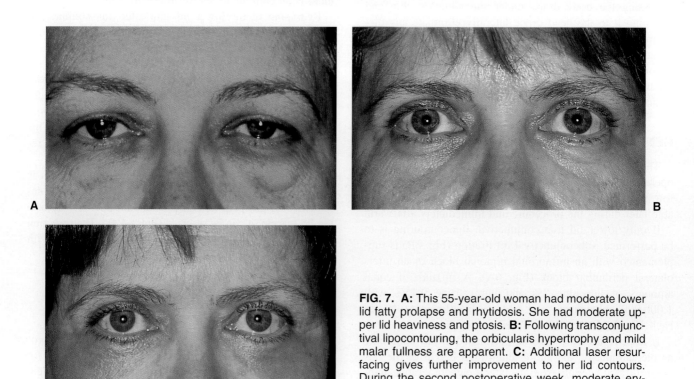

FIG. 7. A: This 55-year-old woman had moderate lower lid fatty prolapse and rhytidosis. She had moderate upper lid heaviness and ptosis. **B:** Following transconjunctival lipocontouring, the orbicularis hypertrophy and mild malar fullness are apparent. **C:** Additional laser resurfacing gives further improvement to her lid contours. During the second postoperative week, moderate erythema and mild edema persist with mild transient secondary lower lid retraction.

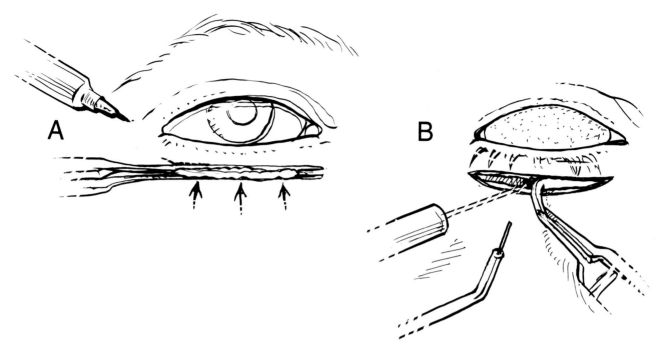

FIG. 8. A: In those exceptionally rare cases of extreme lower lid skin excess 3 months following laser resurfacing, the excess skin is grasped in the lower lid crease and demarcated. **B:** The excess is resected with a CO_2 laser or radiosurgical electrode.

palpebral conjunctiva and the inferior fornix are exposed. Gentle pressure is applied to the globe, causing the prolapsing orbital fat to bulge against the lower lid retractors and palpebral conjunctiva. A disposable cautery, radiosurgical electrode, or 0.2-mm CO_2 laser cutting handpiece in-

cises the conjunctiva over the bulge midway between the inferior tarsal margin and the inferior fornix (Fig. 9A,B).

Additional gentle pressure on the globe and the resultant bulge identifies the area of lower lid retractors overlying the prolapsing fat. The lower lid retractors are incised cen-

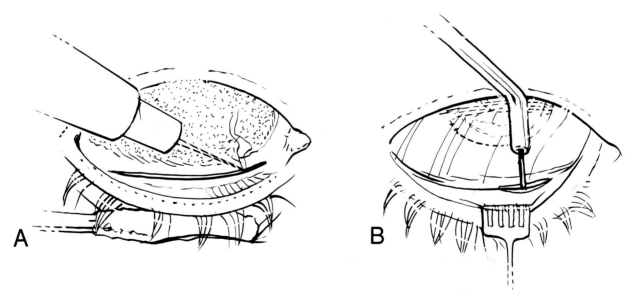

FIG. 9. A,B: The lower lid margin is retracted. Gentle pressure is applied to the globe, causing the fat to bulge. The palpebral conjunctiva is incised midway between the inferior tarsal border and the inferior fornix, over the bulge using a CO_2 laser **(A)** or a radiosurgical electrode **(B)**.

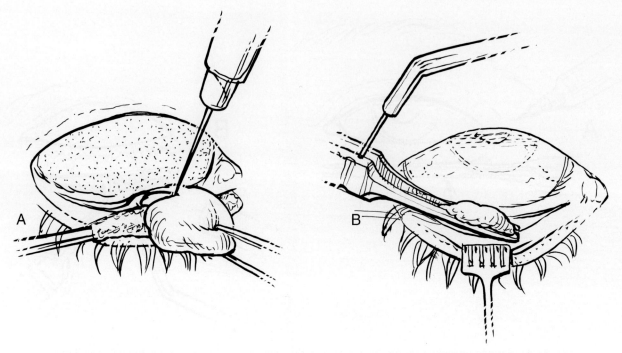

FIG. 10. A: Prolapsing orbital fat is transected with a CO_2 laser while it is supported over a moistened cotton-tipped applicator. **B:** If radiosurgery is employed for fat resection, any blood vessels or the base of the fat resection are grasped with a forceps and the electrode is touched to the forceps.

trally over the bulge. The prolapsing central fat pocket is resected or vaporized until the anterior lower lid contour is acceptable by palpation, while gentle pressure is applied to the globe (Fig. 10A,B). The palpebral conjunctival and lower lid retractor incisions are extended nasally to expose the inferior oblique and nasal fat pockets and then temporally to expose the lateral fat pocket. In turn, each fat pocket is resected or vaporized.

When resection is complete, the lower lid margin is pulled superiorly while the inferior sulcus is massaged with the surgeon's finger. This reduces the possibility of postoperative adhesions of the lower lid retractors. The conjunctiva is not sutured.

FAT PAD RESECTION

Three fat pads—medial, middle, and lateral—have been described in the lower lid. Although they are contiguous in the deep orbit, drawing on the same deep orbital adipose reservoir, these fatty pockets may appear as discrete and separate entities (Fig. 11). Convex protuberances, these fat pockets are separated by fascial septa when they prolapse anteriorly. Abduction will accentuate the nasal pocket. Adduction will accentuate the temporal pocket. Supraduction will accentuate the inferior pockets. These maneuvers will not accentuate convexities secondary to lid edema. Familial-predisposition, septal weakness, or true septal hernias may be responsible for anterior fatty prolapse and secondary lid contour abnormalities. Preoperative annotation of

the location and extent of fat pad prolapse is essential, since the fat pockets may not be as evident with the patient supine on the operating table (Fig. 12A,B).

Fat pad prolapse can affect each compartment individually or collectively. The central and nasal fat pockets are separated by the inferior oblique muscle. The central and lateral fat pockets are separated by the arcuate expansions

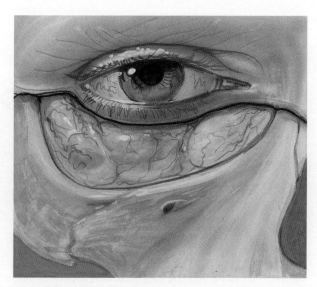

FIG. 11. The three lower lid fat pockets may appear as separate entities.

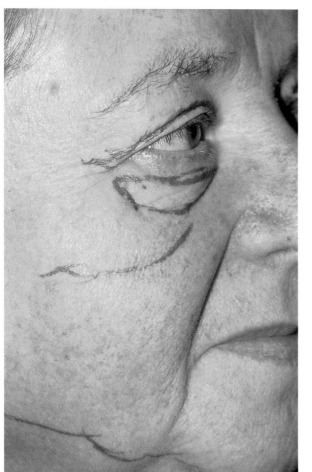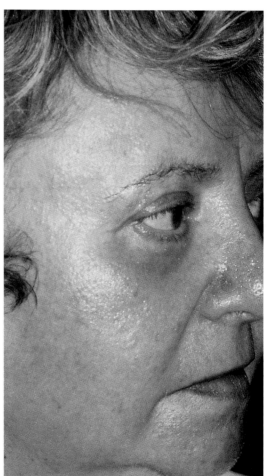

A   B

FIG. 12. A: Lower lid fatty prolapse and malar fullness are delineated on this 56-year-old woman preoperatively before she enters the operating suite. **B:** Three weeks following lower and upper lid recontouring and full-face laser resurfacing, her eyelid and facial contours are improved. Mild erythema persists.

of the inferior oblique. Temporal fat pad prolapse may be problematic. Unless the lid incision is extended sufficiently temporally, this fat pad will not be completely resected and will leave a residual deformity. A secondary deep temporal fat pad may exist posterior to the superficial pad. The unwary surgeon may find postoperatively that the lid bulge that he or she and the patient had studied preoperatively remains insufficiently improved after surgery. After removal of the superficial temporal fat pad, additional attempts to prolapse the secondary pad are essential for satisfactory results.

The surgeon has a choice of methods of fat resection and sculpting. Clamping prolapsed orbital fat, transecting it, and cauterizing the stump has long been the accepted, safe technique (Fig. 13). It is still useful in patients when hemostasis is a problem, but we have largely disregarded clamping-cutting-cauterizing in favor of more accurate, less traumatic open-sky techniques utilizing radiosurgery or a CO_2 laser.

Disposable battery-operated cauteries that are hot enough to cauterize large blood vessels within the orbital fat can

be used, but care must be taken not to ignite the eyelashes. Unipolar electric cauteries supply enough heat to provide complete hemostasis at the base of resected fat, but the patient must be grounded, and there is the theoretical potential of having current conducted through the optic nerve or of burning the patient at the grounding site. Bipolar electric cauteries that require no grounding and do not spark can also be used (Fig. 14).

CLAMPING-CUTTING-CAUTERIZING

The lower lid retractors are opened over the bulge. Gentle pressure is applied to the globe. After the bright yellow central fat pocket mushrooms, its base may be clamped with a curved hemostat. The fat is shaved off the anterior convex surface of the clamp. If the patient is being given nasal oxygen, it must be turned off before the cautery or laser is used. A spark may ignite the patient's eyebrows, eyelashes, or nasal hairs. Electric cautery (set at an appropriate level to mildly char but not to spark) or a radiosurgical electrode is touched to the

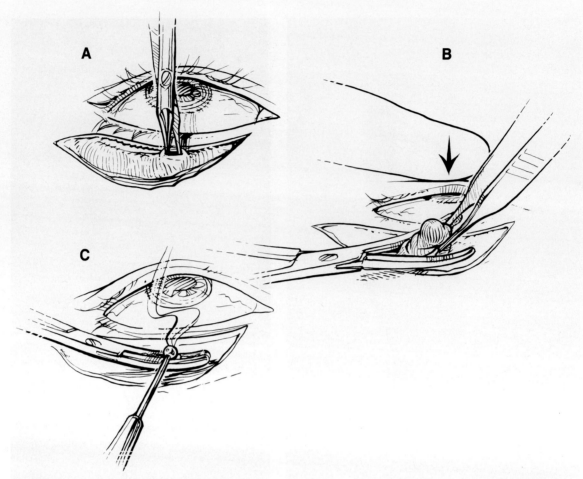

FIG. 13. We rarely use the techniques of transcutaneous lower lid blepharoplasty and clamping, cutting, and cauterizing of the fat pockets.

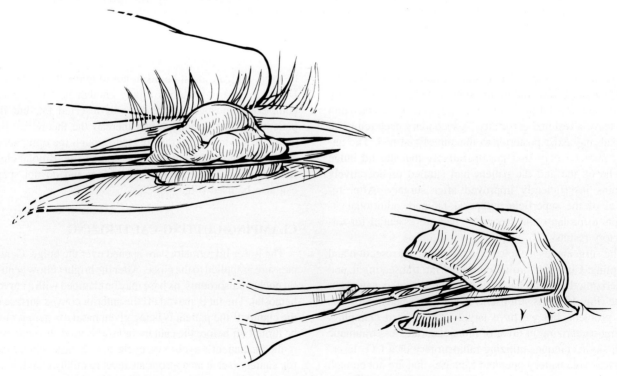

FIG. 14. Prolapsing orbital fat is grasped with a bipolar forceps. This will reduce the size of the fatty bulge, which can then be trimmed along the cauterized margin.

clamped surface of the base of the fat pad. Care is taken to avoid touching cautery or clamp to the lid margin. The base of the fat pad is grasped with a toothed Adson forceps before the clamp is released. If any bleeders are identified, they can be reclamped and cauterized before they retract into the deep orbit (see Fig. 13).

Gentle pressure is again applied to the globe. Any recurrent fatty prolapse is clamped, cut, and cauterized. In a similar fashion, the retractors are incised over the fat bulges, and the lateral and nasal fat pockets are exposed, clamped, cut, and cauterized. The fat from the nasal pocket is much whiter, thicker in texture, and more vascular than that from the other pockets. Fat is never aggressively teased or pulled out of the orbit; this maneuver may increase the potential for retrobulbar hemorrhage and can produce a deep inferior sulcus.

OPEN-SKY RESECTION

The lower lid conjunctiva and retractors are opened widely, exposing the anterior surface of each of the fat pads. The prolapsed fat is grasped with toothed Adson forceps and stabilized as gentle pressure is applied to the globe, accentuating fatty prolapse. Wesscott scissors, a disposable cautery, a radiosurgery electrode, or a 0.2-mm CO_2 laser handpiece is used to release the septal adhesions and sculpt the fat without clamping it.

Large vessels are easily visualized and can be clamped and cauterized, grasped with a forceps, and obliterated with a radiosurgery electrode or a defocused 0.2-mm CO_2 laser handpiece, when they are encountered. These vessels are more commonly found nasally. The sequence of gentle bulbar pressure and fat trimming is streamlined and achieves greater accuracy without the intervening steps of clamping and cauterizing. The complete visualization of the fat pockets makes this a safe and effective technique.

MALAR FESTOONS

Malar festoons are deformities that have been most difficult to correct in the past (Fig. 15). Standard blepharoplasty techniques alone have not been adequate. The CO_2 laser has added another approach.

Excessive redundancy of lower lid skin and orbicularis that cascades below the inferior orbital rim is not amenable to resection via a subciliary lid incision (Fig. 16A–D). Historically, a subciliary lower lid blepharoplasty incision with extensive subcutaneous undermining beyond the inferior orbital rim characteristically leaves a postoperative pocket of subcutaneous edema and residual redundancy over the malar eminence. Injection of these residual inflammatory festoons with methylprednisolone acetate (Depo-Medrol) may minimize the deformity. Extensive undermining of a skin–muscle flap with periosteal anchoring at the lateral palpebral raphe and internal suspension of malar suborbicularis fat to the inferior orbital rim has been described to

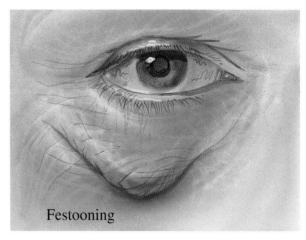
Festooning

FIG. 15. Before the cosmetic use of the CO_2 laser, malar festoons were exceedingly difficult to correct.

eliminate the festoons (Fig. 17A–C). A rhytidectomy with SMAS (Subcutaneous Musculo-aponeurotic System) (Ellman International, Hewlett, NY) plication and extensive skin undermining will supply additional superiorly directed support to the lid–cheek complex and may also minimize malar redundancy. CO_2 laser resurfacing of the malar festoon can significantly reduce mild to moderate deformities; two or three passes using maximum power are usually necessary (Fig. 18; see also Fig. 12).

Residual malar festoons are corrected with direct resections (Fig. 19A,B). Direct inframalar resection of the festoons effectively eliminates the redundancy but leaves the patient with an uncamouflaged scar that in most instances will have to be resurfaced with the CO_2 laser.

The malar festoons are demarcated with methylene blue, and the nasal and temporal edges are tapered, delineating an elliptical resection (Fig. 19A). The vertical expanse of the resection is pinched with toothed Adson forceps, and the lower lid margin is observed to ensure that the resection will not distort the lower lid margin. Lidocaine 2% with 1:200,000 epinephrine is injected subcutaneously in the area of proposed resection. The demarcated festoon incision is incised, and the demarcated area is resected. Underlying premalar and inframalar fat pockets may then be resected. The area is resurfaced with a CO_2 or Er:YAG laser. The wound is closed with interrupted 6-0 nylon sutures (Fig. 19B).

MALAR BAGS

Anecdotal history describes a separate fat pocket at or below the level of the malar eminence. If it is contiguous with the postseptal fat, it can be recontoured via a transconjunctival approach. It may or may not be associated with festoons of skin and orbicularis muscle. As with malar festoons, correction may be attempted with extensive un-

(text continues on page 82)

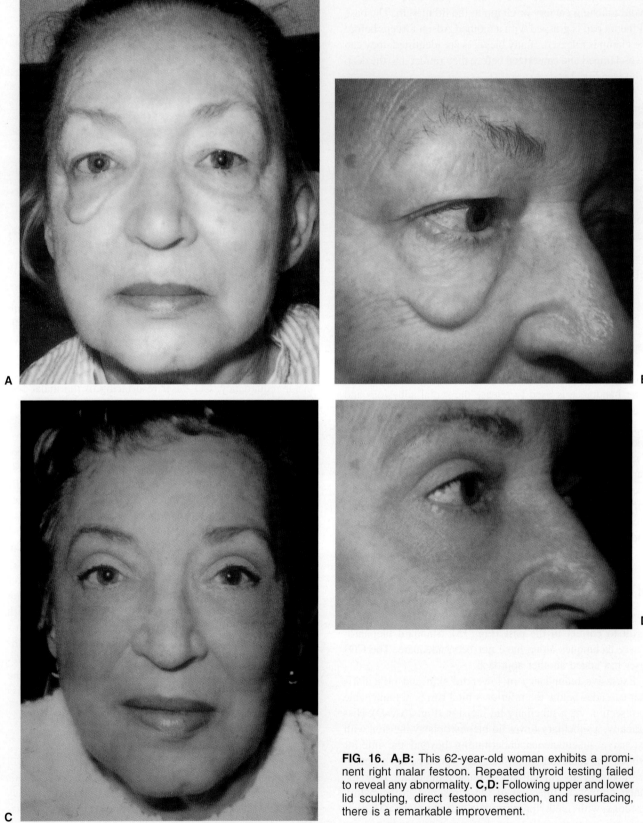

FIG. 16. A,B: This 62-year-old woman exhibits a prominent right malar festoon. Repeated thyroid testing failed to reveal any abnormality. **C,D:** Following upper and lower lid sculpting, direct festoon resection, and resurfacing, there is a remarkable improvement.

LOWER LIDS: ANATOMY AND SURGICAL TECHNIQUES / 81

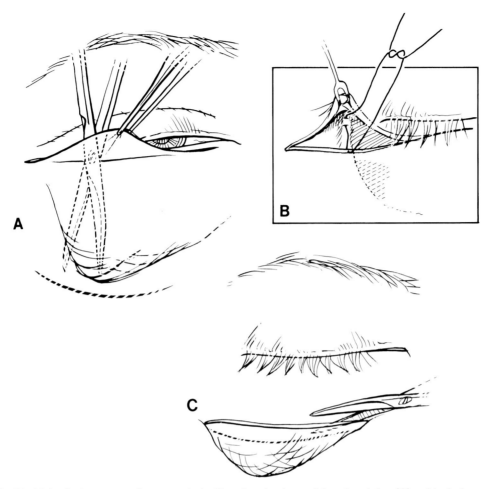

FIG. 17. Malar festoons may be corrected with extensive lower lid undermining (A), orbicularis muscle suspension to the lateral orbital rim (B), and direct resection (C). Internal suspension of the malar suborbicularis fat to the inferior orbital rim can also be employed.

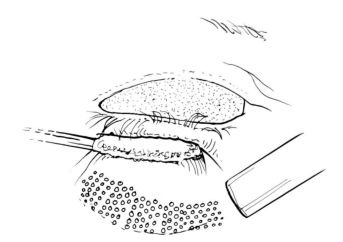

FIG. 18. Heavy laser resurfacing of the malar area may correct mild to moderate malar thickening.

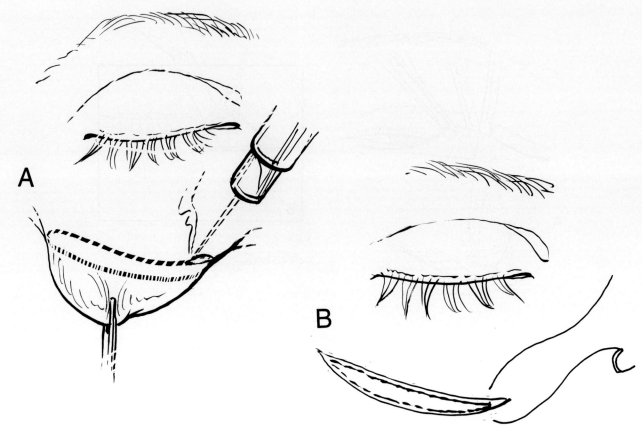

FIG. 19. A,B: Laser resurfacing following direct malar resection is necessary in more marked instances. The malar festoons are demarcated. The nasal and temporal edges are tapered. The amount to be resected is grasped with forceps to avoid displacement of the lower lid margin.

dermining from a subciliary incision, but direct elliptical resection of the redundant malar skin or a direct malar incision for fat resection only is more effective under most circumstances. This deformity may not be amenable to CO_2 laser resurfacing. The major drawback remains the separate incision and scar over the malar eminence that will then need laser resurfacing.

LOWER LID HORIZONTAL LAXITY WITH OR WITHOUT FRANK ECTROPION

Laxity of the lower lid, allowing it to be passively stretched more than 6 mm from the anterior surface of the globe, may predispose the lid to postoperative eversion or retraction of the lid margin. This was particularly relevant in the era of transcutaneous lower lid blepharoplasty. The transconjunctival approach, however, minimizes the risk of lower lid margin displacement, but any lower lid margin laxity must be addressed before lower lid resurfacing is performed.

Correction of Mild to Moderate Lower Lid Margin and Canthal Tendon Laxity: Lateral Canthal Plication

The majority of blepharoplasty patients who have some degree of laxity of the lower lid margin can be corrected with this procedure. It is minimally invasive and effective, and leaves the lateral canthal angle and the lateral palpebral raphe intact. It is an excellent prophylactic technique for patients with borderline lower lid laxity who are undergoing lower lid resurfacing.

A 4-mm lateral upper lid crease incision overlying the lateral orbital rim is made. The periosteum of the orbital rim is exposed (Fig. 20A). A 2-mm lateral lower lid subciliary incision is made. A double-armed mattress suture of 4-0 Prolene is passed from the lower lid palpebral conjunctiva through the subciliary incision. Each arm of the suture is again passed into the subciliary incision, directed laterally and superiorly, engaging the lateral canthal tendon and exiting through the upper lid crease incision. Each arm of the suture is then anchored to the periosteum of the lateral orbital rim. The suture is tied and tightened until the lid margin is in proper apposition to the globe (Fig. 20B). The skin incisions are closed.

Correction of Lateral Canthal Tendon Laxity: Lateral Tarsal Strip

A subtle rounding of the lateral canthal angle or mild S-shaped deformity of the lower lid with a slightly increased vertical palpebral aperture temporally is indicative of lateral canthal tendon laxity. Nasal traction on the lower lid margin

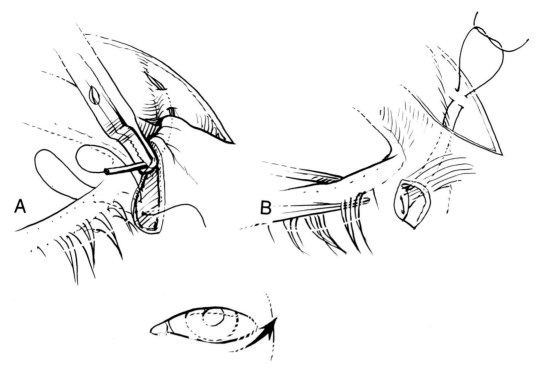

FIG. 20. A: A 4-0 Prolene suture is used to plicate the lateral canthal tendon. It is passed from the palpebral conjunctiva via a lateral subciliary incision, then engaging the tendon; it is anchored to the periosteum of the lateral orbital rim. **B:** The suture is tightened until the lid margin is in proper apposition to the globe.

that narrows the horizontal palpebral aperture and brings the lateral canthal angle closer to the temporal limbus is the result of a markedly lax lateral canthal tendon (Fig. 21A). If the laxity is marked, it will not be corrected with a canthal plication.

A 10- to 12-mm horizontal incision is made over the lateral palpebral raphe from the lateral canthal angle to the lateral orbital rim. A lateral canthotomy is performed with a radio-surgery electrode or a 0.2-mm CO_2 laser handpiece. The inferior crus of the lateral canthal tendon and its periosteal insertion 5 mm posterior to the lateral orbital rim at Whitnall's orbital tubercle are exposed with blunt and sharp dissection. The inferior crus of the lateral canthal tendon is severed from its periosteal insertion. The disinserted lower lid is pulled temporally and notched where it overlaps the lateral orbital rim. The lid margin and lash line are resected temporal to the notch. A base-up triangular resection of orbicularis muscle, lid retractors, and conjunctiva is performed inferior to the tarsus and temporal to the lid margin notch. A tarsal strip is preserved (Fig. 21B). Any tarsus that can be advanced temporally beyond the orbital rim is resected.

At this time, a transconjunctival blepharoplasty of the lower lid may be performed before refixation of the lateral canthal tendon. A double-armed 4-0 Prolene suture is inserted through the tarsal strip 4 mm nasal to its temporal edge. Each arm of this double-armed suture is tunneled laterally beneath the periosteum posterior to the lateral orbital rim, as near Whitnall's lateral orbital tubercle as possible,

and then superiorly through the superior crus of the lateral canthal tendon, exiting superiorly and laterally over the lateral orbital rim (Fig. 21C). Tightening this mattress suture should bring the lower lid into proper apposition with the globe, sharpening the lateral canthal angle, raising the level of the lower lid temporally, and perhaps widening the horizontal palpebral aperture slightly.

Medial Canthal Tendon Laxity

The medial canthal region is an area fraught with great anatomic complexity. Surgery in this area is difficult and should be reserved for those surgeons with familiarity with the anatomic details, technical difficulties, and unique intraoperative hazards. In the absence of frank medial ectropion or punctal eversion, a lax medial canthal tendon may be discovered with the application of lateral traction to the lower lid margin. In the presence of a lax medial canthal tendon, this maneuver will displace the inferior punctum temporally toward the nasal limbus. Clinically significant medial canthal tendon laxity most commonly occurs with long-standing facial palsy—the result of gravity's triumph over an atonic lid. To avoid shortening of the horizontal palpebral aperture, the medial canthal tendon must be plicated before horizontal shortening of the lower lid is performed by wedge resection. Because of the superficial insertion of the anterior lead of the medial canthal tendon and the thin medial canthal skin, there is little opportunity to

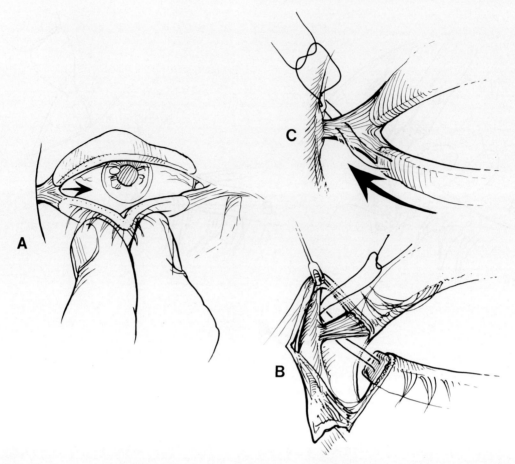

FIG. 21. A: Lateral canthal tendon laxity is confirmed if pinching the lower lid margin narrows the horizontal palpebral aperture and brings the lateral canthal angle closer to the temporal limbus. **B:** After horizontal shortening of the lower lid, preserving a strip of tarsus, the lateral tarsal strip is anchored to the superior crus of the lateral canthal tendon and the periosteum behind the lateral orbital rim. **C:** Plicating a lax lateral canthal tendon will correct mild laxity.

bury the plicating suture. Plication of the medial canthal tendon, even under the best of circumstances, may leave a slight medial canthal bulge with potential to form a suture granuloma—temporarily painful and cosmetically unacceptable. The indications for incorporating this procedure into cosmetic blepharoplasty are limited to marked instability of the inferior punctum and nasal lid margin.

A 12-mm vertical skin incision is demarcated over the periosteal insertion of the medial canthal tendon, beginning above the tendon and extending inferior to it, infiltrated subcutaneously, and incised 10 minutes after infiltration. Dissection with Wesscott scissors, a radiosurgery electrode, or a 0.2-mm CO_2 laser handpiece, while the wound edges are retracted with small rakes, will expose the well defined white tendon approximately 5 mm in width. A suborbicularis muscle tunnel is developed joining the nasal end of the subciliary lid incision. The tendon is plicated in two segments. The origin of the medial canthal tendon and the extreme nasal end of the pretarsal orbicularis are sutured with a double-armed 4-0 Prolene or PDS suture. Each arm of this suture is brought

from the undersurface of the medial canthal tendon at the medial canthal angle through the tendon, exiting on the tendon's anterior surface. A surgeon's knot is tied. The medial canthal tendon is thus plicated and stabilized at two points, securing its position and producing a less obvious bulge.

Although this technique seems straightforward and simple, the exact placement of this suture requires considerable expertise.

Correction of Marked Lower Lid Horizontal Laxity: Wedge Resection

Lower lid margin full-thickness wedge resections are only indicated in cases of extreme lower lid margin laxity that is not corrected with lateral canthal plication or a lateral tarsal strip.

Lidocaine 2% with 1:200,000 epinephrine is injected subcutaneously for the full length and height of the lower lid, extending from as far nasally as the inferior punctum, as far superiorly as the lower lid lash line, and as far inferiorly as the inferior orbital rim. Topical tetracaine is applied to both eyes, and a protective opaque corneal-scleral lens is placed before each of the corneas. The patient is prepared and draped in the usual fashion. A subciliary incision is made along the temporal one-third of the lower lid and 2 mm inferior to the lateral palpebral raphe. If the surgeon has difficulty with countertraction while performing the subsequent skin undermining and developing of a skin flap, a 4-0 black silk suture can be placed in and out of the gray line in the midline of the lower lid and clamped to the sterile drapes superiorly, keeping the lower lid on maximum stretch while stabilizing the lid margin. Toothed Adson forceps are then used to grasp the skin edge and begin the dissection of the skin flap. This is continued and completed, undermining the skin flap as far nasally as the inferior punctum and as far inferiorly as the inferior orbital rim. A short, sharp, straight iris scissors is then used to complete the subciliary incision as far nasally as the inferior punctum. Small rakes are used to retract the skin flap, re-

vealing the underlying pretarsal and preseptal orbicularis muscles.

If there is no canthal tendon laxity, an inverted pentagonal resection of the lower lid is performed at the junction between the temporal one-third and medial two-thirds of the lower lid margin (Fig. 22A,B). A full-thickness lid incision extending from the lid margin to just inferior to the inferior tarsal border is performed with Wesscott scissors. Forceps are then used to grasp the nasal and temporal severed ends of the lid margin and to overlap the ends of the wound and determine the width of the resection (the temporal edge is pulled nasally, and the nasal edge is pulled temporally). The protective corneal-scleral lens is removed to ensure proper apposition of the lid to the globe, without the deforming effect of the protective lens. When the lid is in tight apposition with the globe, the nasal segment of the lid is notched with Wesscott scissors at the point where it overlaps the temporal edge (Fig. 22C,D). The inverted pen-

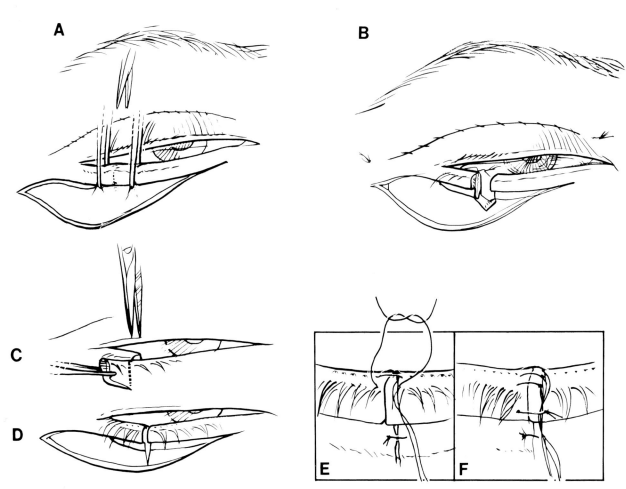

FIG. 22. A: Horizontal shortening of the lower lid margin is performed at the junction of the temporal one-third and nasal two-thirds. **B:** An inverted, pentagonal, wedge-shaped resection will facilitate accurate lid margin anastomosis. **C,D:** The width of the resection is determined by overlapping the severed edges until the lid margin is in proper apposition with the globe. **E,F:** The lid margin is repaired with three interrupted 6-0 black silk sutures placed through the meibomian orifices, the gray line, and the lash line. The suture ends are left long and incorporated under the anterior lamellar sutures.

tagonal resection is then completed and hemostasis is obtained with direct pressure.

The lid margin is reapproximated with a series of 6-0 silk sutures (Fig. 22E,F). The lash line and meibomian line are easily identified and reapproximated, each with a 6-0 black silk suture. The sutures are placed from the second meibomian orifice on either side of the incision of the lid margin. The ends of the sutures are left long so that they can be fixated anteriorly away from the cornea and can also be used for traction. Once the meibomian orifice and lashes have been reapproximated, these sutures can be used for traction and the intervening gray line can be reapproximated with a third 6-0 black silk suture. The tarsus and conjunctiva are closed in one layer with interrupted 5-0 chromic sutures. Overaggressive tightening may accentuate lower lid retraction, inferior scleral show, and rounding of the lateral canthal angle as the lid is pulled below the anterior curvature of the globe.

LOWER LID MALPOSITION—ENTROPION

Involutional entropion of the lower lids can be repaired concomitantly with lower lid blepharoplasty. In the majority of cases, patients have at least a moderate degree of lower lid horizontal laxity. Canthal tendon laxity must be identified and corrected before any horizontal lid shortening procedures are performed.

Our preferred procedure in cases of lower lid entropion is lateral canthal plication with lower lid marginal rotation. In patients with marked horizontal laxity, a lateral tarsal strip or a full-thickness wedge resection can be added.

After a transconjunctival blepharoplasty is performed, the lid margin is everted with a series of mattress sutures of 4-0 chromic. These sutures are equally spaced in the lower lid. The sutures are placed from the palpebral conjunctiva and exit on the skin surface of the lid just anterior to the cilia. The sutures are placed from the inferior fornix and angled superiorly within the lid substance and anteriorly. When the inferior border of the tarsus is reached, the sutures take a more anterior direction. The point of their exit will be determined by the amount of lid margin rotation desired. If the entropion is severe, more lid margin rotation is required. This is accomplished by having the sutures exit more superiorly, closer to the lashes. The second arm of the mattress suture is placed in a similar fashion, and the two ends of the suture are tied to each other. The remaining two marginal rotation sutures are placed in a similar fashion. Then the lid margin is tightened with a lateral canthal plication, a lateral tarsal strip, and/or a lid margin wedge resection.

CHAPTER 7

Blepharoplasty in Men

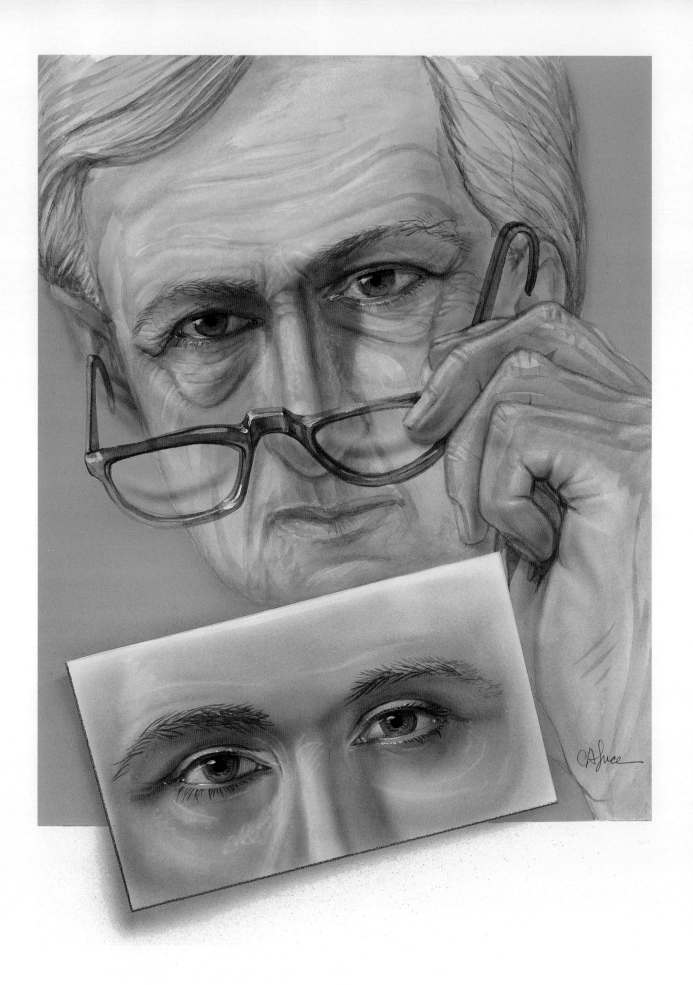

Men can be excellent candidates for cosmetic blepharoplasty, but both the patient and the surgeon must be cognizant of differences in anatomy, technique, and postoperative course from female patients. Men are often less tolerant of postoperative discomfort. Their incisions remain indurated and erythematous for a longer time than those of their female counterparts. Their eyelids may also remain swollen longer.

BROWS

The normal male periocular anatomy differs considerably from the female anatomy. Just as the contour and texture of the male brow differ from the female brow, so do the contour and texture of the upper lids. The low flat contour of the brow parallels a low flat lid fold with minimal central arching. In men, the lid fold is full and generously draped over the lid crease. This is in direct contrast to the deep, smooth female superior sulcus with a high, arched lid crease and a delicate lid fold. Aggressive sculpting of the male superior sulcus and overresecting of the male lid fold are inappropriate. Heavy male upper lid folds and flat brows are accentuated with age. The lid crease, the pretarsal surface, and even the upper lid lashes may be completely obscured. Often, the redundancy may be so great that a levator aponeurotic disinsertion may be completely camouflaged. Frequently accompanying upper lid dermatochalasis and septal weakness in men is brow ptosis, which may be medial, central, or lateral (Fig. 1A,B). The appropriate brow contour should be determined preoperatively. Often, transblepharoplasty internal brow suspension may be all that is necessary.

CORRECTION OF MILD BROW PTOSIS: TRANSBLEPHAROPLASTY INTERNAL SUSPENSION

The procedure that we use most often to correct 1 to 2 mm of lateral brow ptosis with secondary hooding is a transblepharoplasty internal brow suspension. In many men, this is more an internal stabilization rather than a brow elevation. This technique will allow conservative upper lid myocutaneous resection without further lowering of the brow level. Often, this support with minimal elevation will be enough to reduce upper lid fold redundancy in male patients.

An upper lid crease incision is made. A myocutaneous flap is developed. The superior orbital rim is exposed. The brow fat pocket is resected, and the periosteum of the superior orbital rim is exposed (Fig. 2A,B). Internally supporting mattress sutures of 4-0 Prolene anchor the brow to the predetermined level relative to the superior orbital rim. These sutures may be placed segmentally (laterally, centrally, or medially) and may be supplemented with 4-chromic sutures. A strip of lower forehead resurfacing will enhance the result of internal suture suspension (Fig. 3A,B).

CORRECTION OF MODERATE BROW PTOSIS: DIRECT BROWPLASTY WITH FOREHEAD RESURFACING OR ENDOSCOPIC INTERNAL SUSPENSION

In men with a heavy brow and moderate brow ptosis, internal suspension may not be adequate. Direct lateral suprabrow segmental resections and midforehead resections may be employed, followed by laser forehead resurfacing.

A lateral suprabrow full-thickness resection with tapered edges can be used to correct segmental temporal brow ptosis (Fig. 4). The incisions are beveled to avoid transection of brow hair follicles and facilitate wound closure. The length of the incision is determined by the length of the segment to be elevated, and the height of the resection is determined by the amount of elevation required. The interior edge of the muscle resection is anchored to the periosteum with 4-0 Prolene sutures, and the wound is closed with 6-0 nylon. This is followed by laser forehead resurfacing.

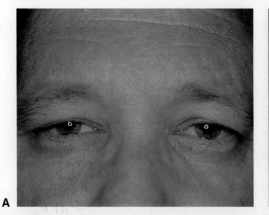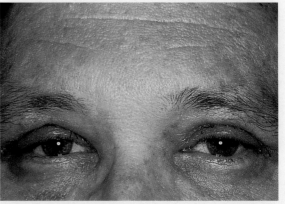

FIG. 1. A: This 55-year-old man had mild brow ptosis and low lid creases. **B:** Minimal myocutaneous resections and internal brow suspensions were used to achieve appropriate brow and upper lid contours.

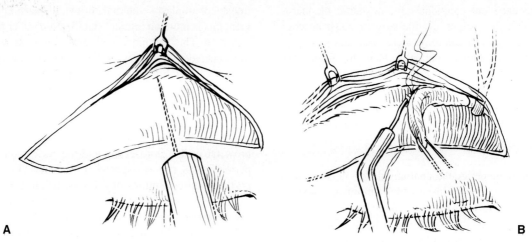

FIG. 2. A: A myocutaneous flap is developed superiorly, exposing the superior orbital rim. **B:** The suborbicularis fat over the superior orbital rim is resected.

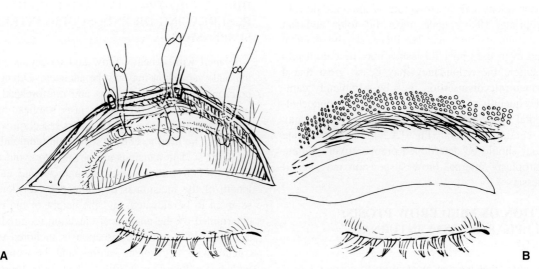

FIG. 3. A: Mattress sutures internally support the brow above the superior orbital rim. **B:** Forehead laser resurfacing can supply additional elevation and support.

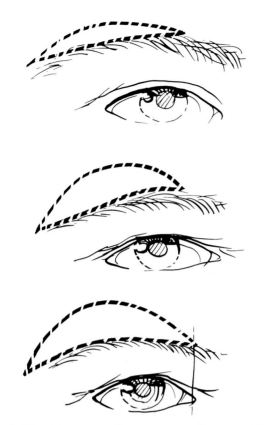

FIG. 4. Direct brow resections can correct segmental temporal brow ptosis.

The transverse forehead furrows can be used in a similar manner to correct medial brow ptosis (Fig. 5) and provide an avenue for resection of the procerus and corrugator muscles (Fig. 6A–C). This can be combined with internal suture stabilization and forehead resurfacing. An endoscopic approach can also be employed.

CORRECTION OF MARKED BROW PTOSIS: BICORONAL APPROACH (SEE CHAPTER 4)

This technique currently has few indications. Most patients find that this procedure sounds too aggressive and do not like the idea of it. And in balding men, as well as men with high foreheads or receding hairlines, its application may be even more limited. However, when brow ptosis is marked, the brows are exceedingly heavy, and other procedures have not been effective, this procedure may be the only remaining option.

UPPER LIDS

As a rule, upper lid blepharoplasty in men should involve more conservative myocutaneous resections and less lipocontouring. Deep superior sulci and high lid creases should be avoided.

The male lid crease should be lower and the lid fold more prominent than in women. This is established with a more

inferior placement of the incision (6 to 8 mm above the lid margin) and a less extensive resection of skin and orbicularis muscle. The incision should be rather straight, with minimal central arching, and should not extended laterally (Fig. 7A–C).

LOWER LIDS

Lower lid blepharoplasty in men may be a complex undertaking for the unwary surgeon. Men with thick, boggy lower lids, heavy howls, and prominent temporal fat pad prolapse often require aggressive transconjunctival fat resection with canthal suspension (Fig. 8) and retractor recession to achieve a smooth lower lid contour without lower lid retraction (Fig. 9A–C).

In selected cases, a concomitant rhytidectomy may be necessary for additional lower lid support.

In younger men without periocular laxity or heaviness of the lower facial musculature, a fine result may be achieved with transconjunctival fat contouring alone.

The transconjunctival lower lid blepharoplasty has greatly simplified the approach to male lower lid blepharoplasty. It minimizes the risk of lower lid retraction, and when combined with lateral canthal plication and stabilization, it will give an adequate margin of safety for performing lower lid laser resurfacing.

Transconjunctival blepharoplasty with lateral canthal suspension and aggressive malar laser resurfacing is an effective technique for treating malar fullness and mild to moderate festooning in men.

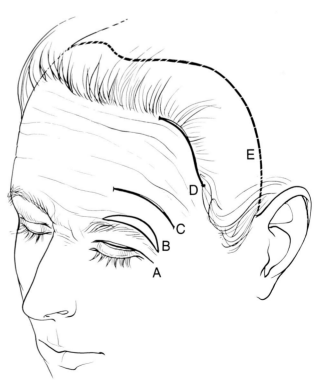

FIG. 5. Transverse forehead furrows (C) can be used for midforehead resections to correct medial brow ptosis.

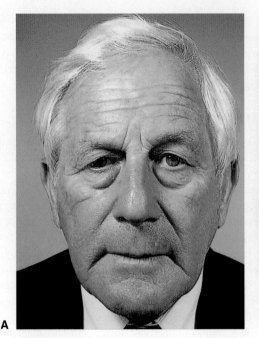

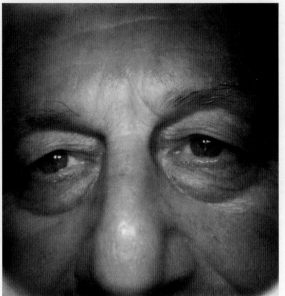

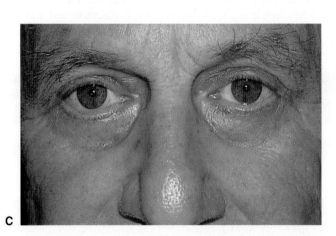

FIG. 6. A: Successful blepharoplasty in men is often more complex than simply resecting redundant lid folds or prolapsed orbital fat. This 68-year-old man had generalized brow ptosis (more marked on the right than the left, with a prominent right-sided medial component). His marked lid fold draping obscured elevated lid creases and levator aponeurotic disinsertions. He also had marked inferior fatty prolapse with moderate lower lid margin laxity. **B:** A close-up view accentuates the narrowed palpebral apertures and lid crease obliterations. **C:** A satisfactory brow elevation with an appropriate, minimally arched male brow contour was obtained with a midforehead lift (his high forehead and receding hairline were contraindications to a coronal scalp flap). His upper lid levels, contours, and creases were reconstructed with skin–muscle resection, fat contouring, and levator aponeurotic repairs. Adequate lower lid contours were achieved, without altering the lower lid levels, with fat contouring, horizontal shortening, and lateral tarsal strip suspensions.

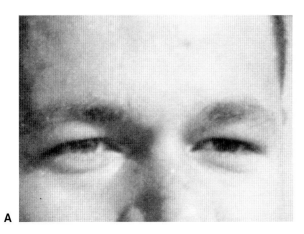

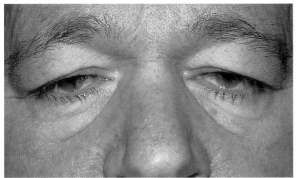

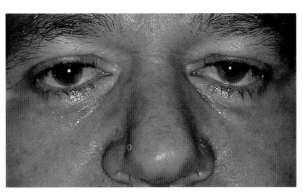

FIG. 7. A: An old photograph is used to help determine the proposed lid and brow levels and contours. **B:** This 55-year-old man had moderate brow ptosis, severe upper lid fullness, moderate blepharoptosis, mild to moderate lower lid fat herniation, and moderate malar fullness. **C:** A natural, youthful result approximating his old photo is achieved with upper lid transblepharoplasty, internal brow suspension, a strip of laser forehead resurfacing, levator aponeurotic advancements, conservative lipocontouring, lower lid transconjunctival lipocontouring, lateral canthal suspension, and lower lid and malar laser resurfacing.

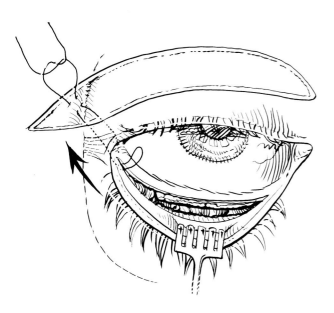

FIG. 8. The technique of transconjunctival lipocontouring with recession of the lower lid retractors and lateral canthal suspensions can correct baggy lower lids and achieve smooth lower lid contours in men without risking lower lid retraction.

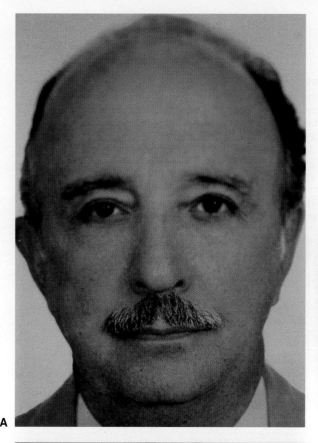

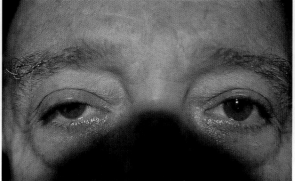

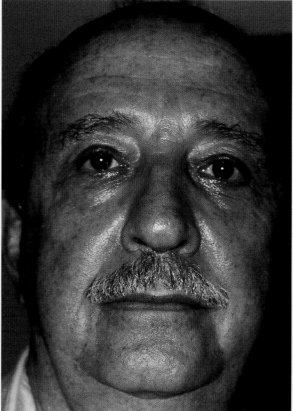

FIG. 9. A: An old photograph of the patient helps us determine the desired lid levels and contours. **B:** This 64-year-old man had bilateral levator aponeurotic disinsertions, ptosis, and moderate to marked lower lid fatty prolapse. **C:** His appearance approximated his old photograph following bilateral levator aponeurotic repairs and transconjunctival lipocontouring.

CHAPTER 8

Blepharoplasty in Asian Patients

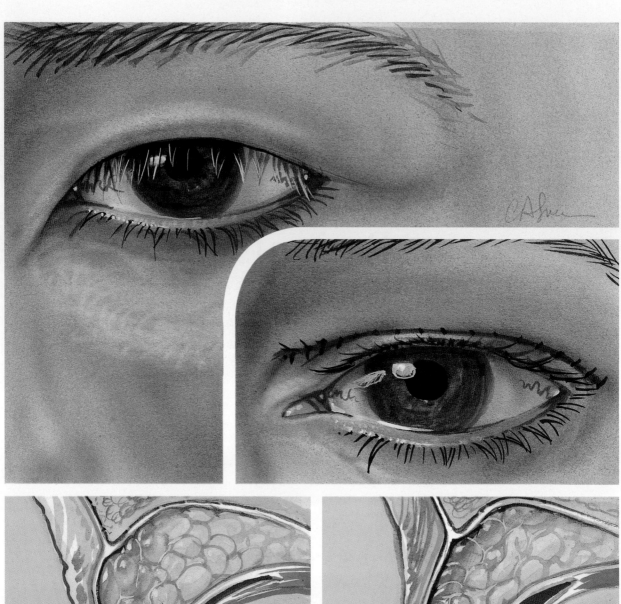
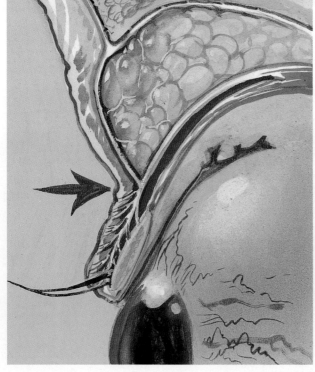
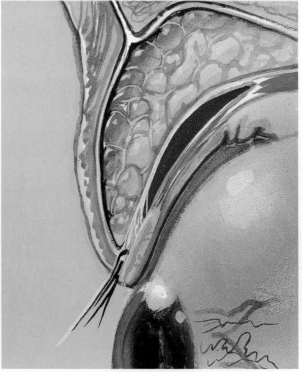

UPPER LID BLEPHAROPLASTY

Because of variation in the upper lid anatomy of Asians, the techniques normally applied to white patients may not yield the desired result. There are three areas of potential concern: the lid crease–fold complex, the epicanthal folds, and the angle and width of the horizontal palpebral aperture.

Most of our Asian patients are particularly attentive to the height, depth, length, and symmetry of their lid crease–fold complexes. They are very specific and exact about their desires and expectations. Even minor alterations must be attempted with great care (Fig. 1A,B). It has also been our impression that patients from different cultures have different aesthetics and different opinions about that they consider attractive in an eyelid. For these reasons, we recommend only subtle, very natural changes in the height and contour of the lid–crease fold complex. We do not recommend deepening of the superior sulcus or changes in the lateral canthal angle.

LID CREASE–FOLD COMPLEX

Perhaps of paramount importance is the lid crease–fold complex. The lid fold has increased prominence in Asian patients for multiple reasons:

- The lid fold often will completely obscure the lid crease. The anterior expansions of the levator aponeurosis, unlike those of Caucasian patients, are weak or nonexistent, or insert far inferiorly near the lid margin (Table 1).
- There can be a less defined or prolapsed preaponeurotic fat pad (pretarsal fat not restrained by the orbital septum), as well as substantial subcutaneous deposition of fat.
- There may be a redundant, lax, ballooned septum with a low insertion onto the tarsus.
- There is usually a significant amount of subcutaneous fat (Fig. 2).

A low lid crease may be evident only when the lid fold is retracted (Fig. 3A,B). The lid crease may not be present at all, or it may occur at a level approximating the lid level in whites. The double eyelid exists when the lid crease is 6 mm or more above the lid margin. When it is less than 4 mm above the margin, it may be perceived as a single eyelid.

There are profound ethnic variations among Chinese, Japanese, Korean, and Filipino patients. The procedure must be individualized for each of these patient populations. Patients must understand that any resection of upper lid skin and orbicularis muscle may create a lid crease and may occidentalize the lid. Many patients specifically want to occidentalize their lids (Fig. 4A–C). Some desire a double eyelid without changing their ethnic character. Others complain of lid heaviness; they want only the excess resected and do not want their appearance changed (Fig. 5A,B). In this latter group are patients with true blepharoptosis who do not want the character of their upper lids to be altered; the skin incisions must be lower, either in a preexisting crease or, if one does not exist, no higher than 4 to 5 mm above the lashes (see Fig. 3A,B). In this group, the septum and preaponeurotic fat should be left intact, if possible.

In patients desiring a double eyelid without occidentalization, the lid crease should be demarcated 4 to 5 mm above the lashes. A skin–muscle resection including preseptal adipose tissue is performed (Figs. 6A, 7A). The septum is opened to the full width of the skin–muscle resec-

(text continues on page 101)

TABLE 1. *Causes of lid fold prominence in single-eyelid Asian patients (lid crease obscuration)*

Inferior insertion of levator aponeurosis
Lack of anterior aponeurotic expansions
Pretarsal fat: redundant or incompetent septum
Subcutaneous fat

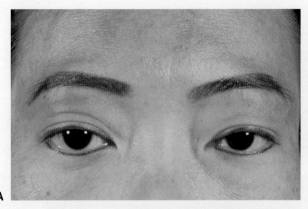 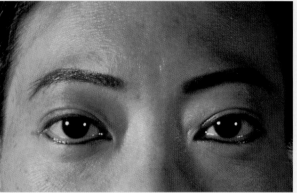

FIG. 1. A: This 32-year-old Japanese woman had asymmetry of her upper lid crease–fold complexes. She had multiple creases of her right upper lid and a low left upper lid crease. **B:** A single right upper lid crease was formed, and the left upper lid crease was elevated.

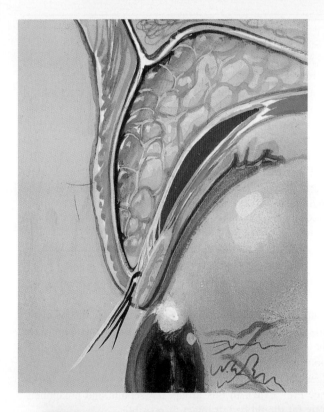

FIG. 2. A ballooned orbital septum with a low insertion onto the levator aponeurosis and lack of anterior insertions onto the skin produce a characteristic Asian upper eyelid with a low or absent lid crease.

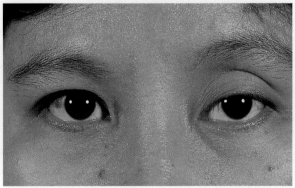 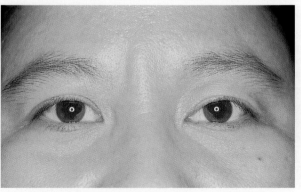

FIG. 3. A: This 27-year-old Filipino woman had a low lid crease of her right upper lid and a retracted left upper lid crease and left upper lid ptosis. The lid crease asymmetry was more striking than her mild ptosis. **B:** Correction of her left upper lid ptosis with a levator aponeurotic advancement via a low lid crease incision reestablished her eyelid symmetry.

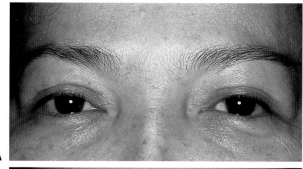
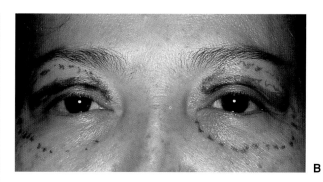
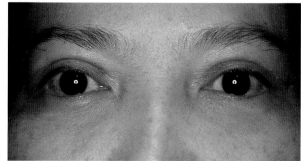

FIG. 4. A: This 34-year-old Chinese woman had previously undergone a lid crease procedure, before coming to our office. She felt that her upper lids were too heavy and her lower lids too baggy. **B:** Conservative lipocontouring of her upper lids without additional skin resection, lower lid transconjunctival lipocontouring, and laser resurfacing were planned. **C:** Following these procedures, there is improvement of her lid contours.

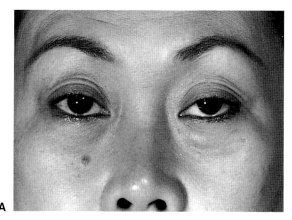
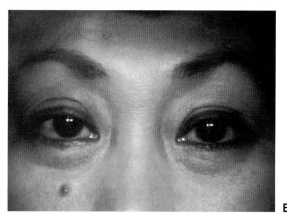

FIG. 5. A: This 40-year-old Filipino woman complained of upper lid heaviness and lower lid fullness. She had upper lid ptosis with lid crease asymmetry and prominent prolapse of her lower lid fat pockets. **B:** Following levator aponeurotic advancement, lid crease reconstruction, and lower lid blepharoplasty, excellent lid levels and contours were achieved without altering her ethnic character.

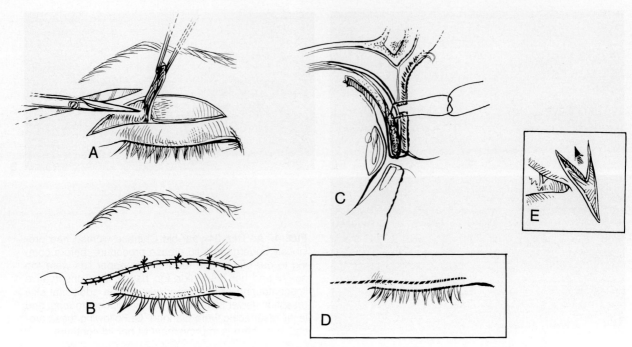

FIG. 6. A: If there is an enlarged lid fold in addition to an absent crease, a skin–muscle resection is performed at the desired level of the lid crease. **B,C:** The lid crease may be formed and the wound closed with sutures incorporating the inferior edge of the levator aponeurosis. **D:** A lower lid crease incision may be used if upper lid resection or ptosis correction is planned without occidentalization. **E:** A V-Y-plasty may be used to diminish epicanthus tarsalis.

FIG. 7. Formation of a lid crease. **A:** Myocutaneous resection. **B:** CO_2 laser contraction of preaponeurotic and subcutaneous fat and orbital septum. **C:** Wound closure incorporating levator aponeurotic insertion.

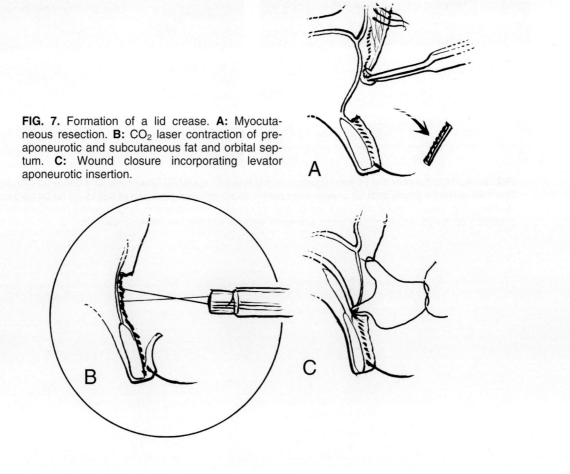

tion. Gentle pressure applied to the globe encourages fat to prolapse and is conservatively resected or vaporized with a carbon dioxide (CO_2) laser (Fig. 7B). Any large vessels are cauterized or vaporized. The levator aponeurosis is visualized. To provide a flat pretarsal contour and avoid reduplication of the lid crease, a 4-mm strip of the superior pretarsal orbicularis is resected. This maneuver may disinsert the inferior edge of the levator aponeurosis. The inferior aponeurotic edge is fixed to the anterior tarsal surface at its midheight with three interrupted 6-0 black silk sutures (Figs. 6B, 7C). The patient is asked to open and close the eyes to confirm the maintenance of the proper lid level and contour.

The wound is closed with a continuous locking 6-0 nylon suture after 6-0 black silk cardinal sutures quadrisect the wound, incorporating the inferior edge of the reinserted levator aponeurosis in the closure (Fig. 6B,C).

Except in patients completely lacking an upper lid crease, we no longer use full-thickness absorbable mattress sutures to form a lid crease. Creases formed in this fashion will remain deep, even on downward gaze, and may look unnatural.

EPICANTHAL FOLDS

Epicanthal tarsalis is the most characteristic fold in northern Chinese and Korean patients. There is a defined lid crease laterally but none nasally, since the fold obscures the nasal lid margin. If the patient wants a more visible lid crease nasally, epicanthus tarsalis can be altered by extending the nasal extent of the upper lid blepharoplasty incision beyond the superior punctum, following the contour of the epicanthal fold. The wound is closed in a V-Y-plasty with interrupted 6-0 black silk sutures (Fig. 6E).

Since Asian patients may have a greater propensity for hypertrophic scarring, medial canthal fold revision should be approached with great caution and the prerequisites of great experience and long-term follow-up.

The epicanthal fold in epicanthus supraciliaris traverses the medial canthus from the eyebrow to the lacrimal sac. The epicanthus palpebralis fold extends from the nasal pretarsal area to the area of the anterior lacrimal crest.

Epicanthus palpebralis and supraciliaris with upper and lower lid components can be modified with double opposing Z-plasties or upper and lower V-Y-plasties.

In the lower lids, a subciliary incision is extended nasal to the inferior punctum, with a V at the extreme nasal end paralleling the inferior aspect of the fold. On suturing of the wound medially, a V-Y-plasty is created.

LATERAL CANTHAL ALTERATIONS

There are profound ethnic variations in lateral canthal angles. If an alteration in the direction of the lateral canthal angle is desired, reinsertion and redirection of the lateral canthal tendon can be attempted.

LOWER LID BLEPHAROPLASTY

Lower lid fatty prolapse is exceedingly common in Asian patients. The transconjunctival approach is well suited for these patients. It avoids the possibility of hypertrophic scarring and alterations in the contour of the palpebral aperture (see Figs. 4A–C, 5A,B).

EYELID RESURFACING

As a rule, Asian patients do not have the profound rhytidosis of the eyelids found in white patients. However, eyelid resurfacing often is still indicated and can be performed successfully (see Fig. 4A–C). When resurfacing is contemplated, preoperative preparation with bleaching agents and alpha-hydroxy acid (AHA) peels is helpful. Patients must be aware that they are likely to experience a transient postoperative period of mottled pigmentation and that after the inflammatory phase has subsided, bleaching agents, AHA peels, and avoidance of sun exposure may be indicated.

CHAPTER 9

Blepharoplasty in Black-skinned Patients

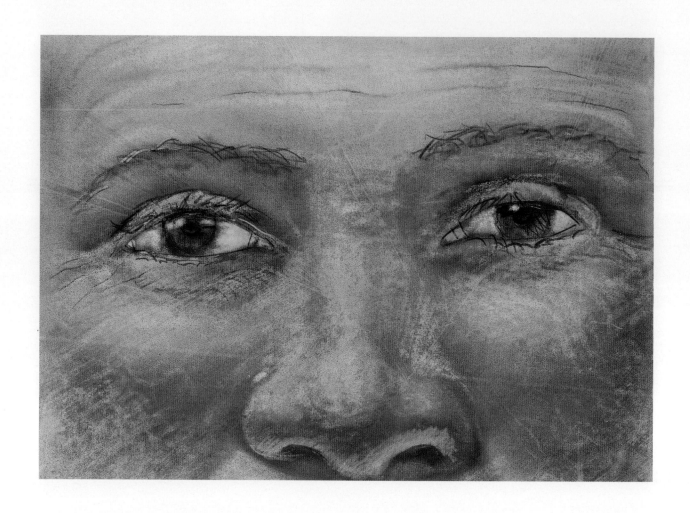

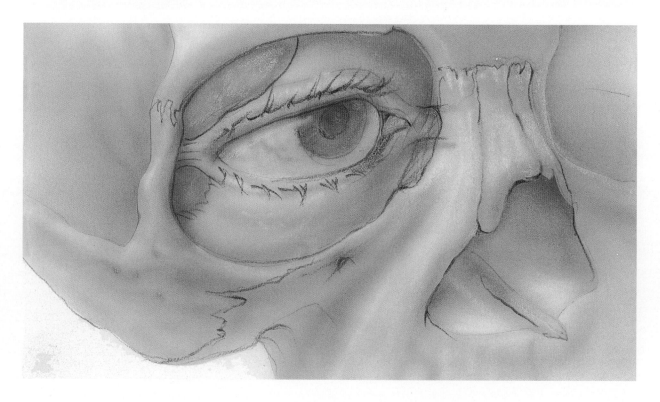

Persons of African descent often have a specific combination of variations of their periocular anatomy that deserve special attention: shallow orbits with prolapsed lacrimal glands and lower lid inferior scleral show (Table 1). Recognizing these variations will increase the likelihood of a successful surgical result (Fig. 1).

UPPER LID BLEPHAROPLASTY

Upper lid temporal fullness is often the hallmark of lacrimal gland enlargement or prolapse. Typically, upper lid blepharoplasty in dark-skinned patients will require more aggressive lipocontouring, sculpting of the brow fat pocket, and repositioning of a prolapsed lacrimal gland (Fig. 2A,B).

Because of the thinness of the upper skin, the possibility of upper lid keloids or hypertrophic scarring is almost nil. A history of keloids on the face or body is not a contraindication to upper lid blepharoplasty (Fig. 3A,B).

LOWER LID BLEPHAROPLASTY

The anatomic complex of shallow orbits, inferior scleral show, and malar hypoplasia can make lower lid blepharoplasty problematic. To avoid lower lid displacement is essential. The transconjunctival approach minimizes the chance of lower lid retraction and obviates a hypertrophic cutaneous cicatrix (Fig. 4A,B).

The shallow orbit and relative malar hypoplasia should alert the surgeon that unless malar augmentation is contemplated, more aggressive lipocontouring will be needed to obtain the desired lower lid contour. Because the globe often sits far anterior to the lateral orbital rim, plicating the lateral canthal tendon may not adequately elevate the lower lid margin and may even draw the lid margin lower. In patients with marked lower lid retraction and relative proptosis, temporalis fascia suspension of the lower lid and/or lateral orbital rim advancement should be considered. In the majority of patients, the most acceptable alternative is to perform a transconjunctival blepharoplasty and leave the lid margin where it is.

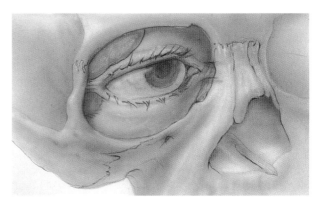

FIG. 1. The characteristic complex periocular anatomy of this patient of African descent includes shallow orbits, prolapsed lacrimal glands, inferior scleral show, relative malar hypoplasia, and relative proptosis.

TABLE 1. *Characteristic complex periocular anatomy in persons of African descent*

Shallow orbit	Relative malar hypoplasia
Prolapsed lacrimal glands	Relative proptosis
Lower lid retraction	

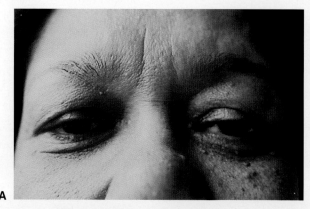
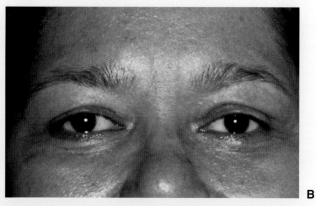

FIG. 2. A: This 46-year-old woman had marked upper lid thickening with temporal fullness, marked lower lid rhytidosis with dermatosis papulosa nigras. **B:** Her lid contours were improved with conservative upper lid myocutaneous resections, lipocontouring, laser lacrimal gland palpebral lobe contouring, and periocular laser resurfacing.

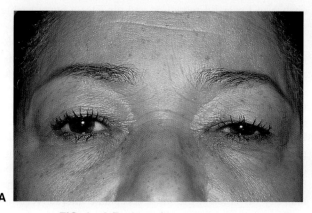
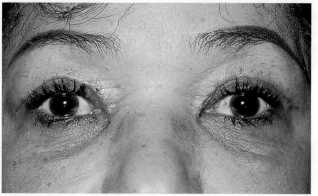

FIG. 3. A,B: Just after suture removal on the sixth postoperative day, this 47-year-old woman shows marked improvement of her lid contours, with little inflammatory response after upper lid myocutaneous resections and lipocontouring and lower lid transconjunctival blepharoplasty.

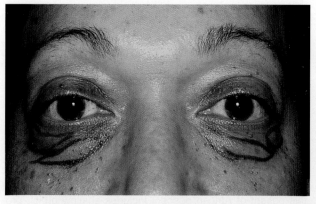
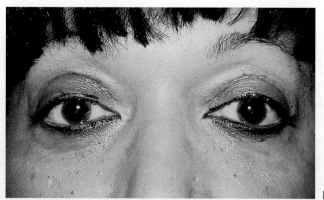

FIG. 4. A: This 45-year-old woman's upper lid temporal fullness is indicative of ptotic or enlarged lacrimal glands. She has prominent eyes and slight temporal retraction of her lower lids. **B:** Following blepharoplasty with laser contraction of the palpebral lobe of her lacrimal glands, there is improved definition of her upper lid contours. The transconjunctival approach to her lower lid fat pockets with recession of her lower lid retractors allowed improved lid contour and lid level.

CHAPTER 10

Complications: Diagnosis and Treatment

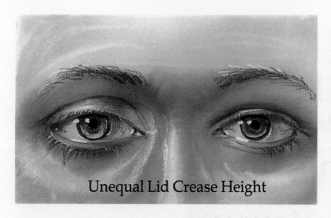

Unequal Lid Crease Height

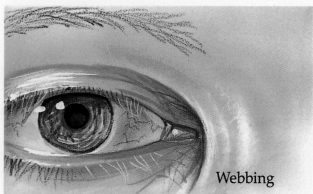

Webbing

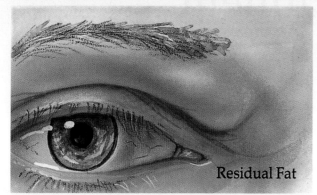

Residual Fat

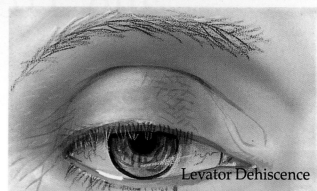

Levator Dehiscence

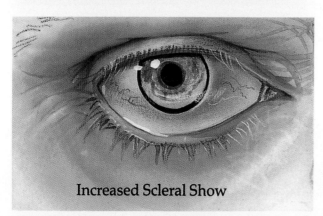

Increased Scleral Show

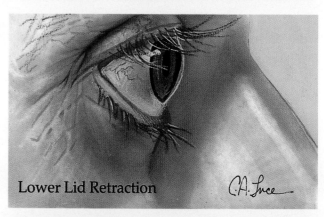

Lower Lid Retraction

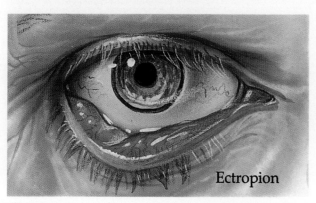

Ectropion

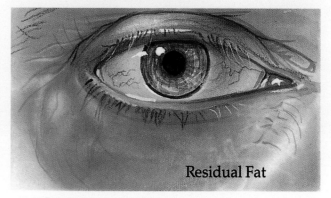

Residual Fat

UPPER LIDS

Suture Tunnels/Inclusion Cysts

Although much is made of suture tunnels, we rarely see them. We leave interrupted 6-0 black silk sutures in place for 5 days. Early suture removal in patients who have had upper lid myocutaneous resections and carbon dioxide (CO_2) laser resurfacing can invite wound dehiscence.

Silk or absorbable sutures left in place for too long may produce small cysts in the suture line. Inclusion cysts along the suture line may be the result of small epithelial remnants left after initial skin incision and later buried in the suture line. We believe that the generous application of ointment to the wound during the first 5 postoperative days will decrease the frequency of these cysts. If they occur, they may be uncapped or marsupialized with a no. 11 blade without local infiltration.

Insufficient Skin Resection

A redundant, objectionable upper lid skin fold following blepharoplasty may be corrected with additional skin–muscle resection or laser resurfacing, if there is no concomitant brow ptosis, medial excess nasal to the superior punctum, lid lag, or lagophthalmos. To convert a good cosmetic result with good lid function to a great cosmetic result with compromised lid function is unwise.

The implementation of eyelid laser resurfacing introduces an additional margin of safety to eyelid rejuvenation. Modifying the amount of upper lid myocutaneous resection and adding laser resurfacing can yield an enhanced cosmetic result with less chance of lid lag or lagophthalmos. Mild residual temporal hooding with a mildly inferiorly displaced brow can be adequately corrected with transblepharoplasty internal suspension.

A moderate residual temporal hooding with a moderately inferiorly displaced brow can be satisfactorily corrected with a direct browplasty. Skin excess nasal to the superior

punctum not adequately resected with a lid crease resection, medial modifications (i.e., W-plasty), or laser resurfacing may need a medial brow elevation for improvement.

Excessive Skin Resection

Our approach to the upper lids—conservative myocutaneous resections and laser resurfacing—has greatly minimized the chances of this complication. Upper lid lag on downward gaze and lagophthalmos on attempted closure are indications of excessive skin resection and anterior lamellar shortening. With marked overresections, the lid crease–fold complex may be obliterated. The tear film and the corneal epithelium may be compromised and necessitate a lifelong regimen of topical lubrication.

Unrecognized brow ptosis may be the cause of overresection of upper lid skin. Repeated lid resections will pull the brows farther inferiorly and create the appearance of residual upper lid skin excess. Subsequent attempts to raise the brows to an appropriate level will accentuate lid lag and lagophthalmos. The remedy is free-skin grafting to supplement the deficient anterior lamella (Fig. 1A–C). Following a blepharoplasty, the best available donor site is retroauricular skin, if a rhytidectomy has not previously been performed. The color, texture, and thickness of retroauricular skin may never exactly match upper lid skin, even after these grafts have been thinned. If there is any question of skin overresection during the initial blepharoplasty surgery, the skin should be wrapped in moist saline gauze and saved in a refrigerator. It may be used as a free-skin graft even 1 week postoperatively.

Upper Lid Retraction

Lid lag, lagophthalmos, and/or superior scleral show can rarely occur without excessive skin resection. They may occur as a result of postoperative fibrosis of the levator aponeurosis (without an obvious cause or secondary to cau-

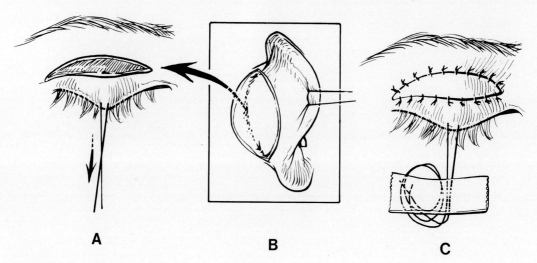

A   **B**   **C**

FIG. 1. A: The previous incision site is incised. A 4-0 black silk traction suture is placed in the gray line, keeping the upper lid on stretch. **B:** A retroauricular graft of the same dimensions is placed into the upper lid defect. **C:** After trimming, the graft edges are anastomosed to the host wound edges. The lid is stabilized with a traction suture fixated to the cheek.

tery to the aponeurosis and septum) or as a result of adhesions between the levator aponeurosis and the orbital septum (secondary to marked postoperative inflammation or excessive intraoperative cautery).

Correction of postblepharoplasty lid retraction requires exploring the wound, releasing all adhesions between the skin–orbicularis layer and the levator aponeurosis and septum, and stretching the lid inferiorly with a traction suture to the malar eminence for 5 to 7 days. Severe, long-standing cases may need recession of the levator aponeurosis with or without a spacer of autogenous temporalis fascia, autogenous fascia lata, tarsus, or auricular cartilage. If there are secondary cicatricial changes of the overlying skin, a retroauricular skin graft may also be necessary.

Ptosis

Transient mechanical ptosis secondary to postoperative lid edema or levator paresis following aggressive fat resection

and cautery will usually resolve without treatment within several weeks. Inadvertent dehiscence of the levator aponeurosis may be caused by resecting a wide band of pretarsal orbicularis muscle (Fig. 2). Immediate direct repair of the levator aponeurotic defect during the surgical procedure is the most effective and predictable technique for correcting postblepharoplasty levator aponeurotic disinsertions. Persistent ptosis without an obvious levator aponeurotic defect should be observed for at least 3 months before surgical repair is attempted. If the ptotic lid is sufficiently elevated after the instillation of two drops of phenylephrine 2.5%, a tarsoconjunctivomüllerectomy with Müller's muscle advancement (Fasanella Servat procedure) may be attempted.

Asymmetric or Inadequate Lid Creases

The lid crease is a prominent surgical and cosmetic landmark. Any lid crease asymmetry in spite of equal palpebral

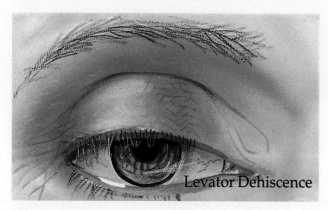

Levator Dehiscence

FIG. 2. Levator aponeurotic disinsertion and ptosis may rarely follow upper lid blepharoplasty.

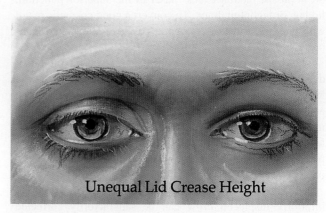

Unequal Lid Crease Height

FIG. 3. Upper lid crease asymmetry may follow upper lid myocutaneous resections.

apertures will be most apparent (Fig. 3). Complete absence of a lid crease within 8 to 12 mm from the lash line denotes either complete disinsertion of the levator aponeurosis or marked deficiency of upper lid skin. Both instances are rare. More commonly, the distance from the upper lid margin to the lid crease may be asymmetric. If there is an adequate amount of residual upper lid skin, it is easier to lower a lid crease than to elevate it. Surgery is performed on the lid with the higher crease. A skin–muscle resection of appropriate height is performed inferior to the crease. The orbicularis muscle ends are reapproximated with the skin closure to establish the crease at a lower level.

Superior Sulcus Asymmetry

Excessive fat resection may create an inappropriately deep superior sulcus. Correction is difficult, but the implantation of fat pearls or the transplantation of fat pedicle flaps have been used with moderate success. In an animal model, hyaluronic acid gel [e.g., Hylaform (Biomatrix, Saint Tropez, France), Restylane (Q Med, Uppsala, Sweden)] has yielded long-term improvement.

Residual upper lid fat may also create superior sulcus asymmetries (Fig. 4).

Extraocular Muscle Imbalance

The trochlea and tendon of the superior oblique muscle may be traumatized during aggressive manipulation of the superior nasal fat pocket and can yield transient diplopia.

Forehead Paresthesias

Disruption of the supratrochlear, infratrochlear, or supraorbital neurovascular bundles may follow aggressive resection of the superior nasal fat pocket. Normal forehead sensation will return in several months.

Suborbicularis browfat pocket resection may also result in transient paresthesia of the temporal brow and forehead.

LOWER LIDS

Hematoma

In the past, gravity and lymphatic drainage made lower lid hematomas more common than upper lid hematomas. Orbicularis muscle and orbital fat were the most common sites for bleeding. Persistent, active postoperative bleeding necessitated opening the wound, localization and cautery of the bleeding site, removal of the hematoma, and resuturing the cutaneous subciliary incision wound. Gradual, self-limited oozing within the orbicularis muscle also produced hematomas.

We have eliminated the transcutaneous lower lid blepharoplasty from our list of proposed surgical options. The transconjunctival lower lid blepharoplasty eliminates the incision of orbicularis muscle and thus reduces postoperative

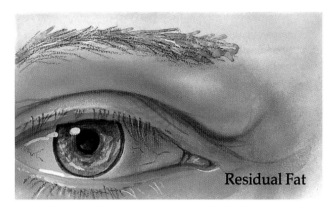

FIG. 4. Residual upper lid fat may create a superior sulcus asymmetry.

ecchymosis and the risk of hematoma. Use of the CO_2 laser with concomitant defocusing for vessel obliteration has substantially reduced the occurrence of postoperative hematomas and virtually eliminated the possibility of postoperative hemorrhage. Although we have never encountered it, if there is significant postoperative bleeding from a sudden elevation in blood pressure, we would open the conjunctival incision and apply cautery to the bleeding site.

Conjunctival Chemosis

Transient conjunctival edema following transconjunctival blepharoplasty may last 2 to 3 days. Longer lasting conjunctival edema may follow a lateral tarsal strip suspension. This may last 2 to 3 weeks and be somewhat ameliorated with steroid drops and lymphatic drainage massage.

Epiphora

Patients complaining of tears welling up around their eyes, tears running down their cheeks, or blurred vision may have excessive lacrimation. This may be secondary to postoperative lid inflammation and edema, with resultant decreased blinking and transient lagophthalmos. If the disturbed blinking patterns have decreased tear breakup times or if compromised lid closure has caused corneal exposure with exposure keratitis and epithelial defects, epiphora may result. The frequent application of tear substitute drops during the day and lubricating ointments at bedtime will relieve the symptoms. An alternative therapy—temporary insertion of punctum plugs—will obviate or supplement topical therapy. All of these symptoms, however, should resolve within 2 to 3 weeks. Persistent complaints after all inflammatory signs have vanished may indicate a structural malposition—punctal eversion, lid retraction, or keratitis sicca.

Punctal Eversion

The elimination of subciliary cutaneous incisions has markedly reduced the occurrence of punctal malposition following lower lid blepharoplasty. Inferior punctal eversion may occur without frank lower lid ectropion. The inferior punctum, normally hidden in the medial lacrimal lake, is strikingly susceptible to mild anterior lamellar cicatricial changes. Punctal eversion may be the result of mild medial skin cicatrization. Any rotation of the punctum out of the lacrimal lake, either verticalization or obvious eversions, may produce epiphora.

During laser resurfacing at the lower lid, it is prudent to avoid the pretarsal skin anterior to the inferior punctum. Mild punctal eversion often may be corrected with massage during the early postoperative period. If punctal displacement is slight, massage may even be continued for 3 months before additional therapeutic measures are suggested.

If there is no improvement of mild to moderate punctal malposition after 3 weeks of massage, minimal or no lid margin horizontal laxity, and minimal or no nasal lid margin retraction on upward gaze, a retropunctal resection of palpebral conjunctiva and submucosal cauterization can be used to rotate the punctum back into the lacrimal lake (Fig. 5). Topical tetracaine is applied to the palpebral and bulbar conjunctiva. Lidocaine 2% with 1:200,000 epinephrine is injected subcutaneously and subconjunctivally inferior and nasal to the punctum. The inferior punctum is dilated with a punctum dilator, and a 00 Bowman probe is inserted into the inferior canaliculus (for retraction and identification).

Four millimeters inferior to the punctum on the palpebral conjunctiva, a transverse conjunctival incision is made, extending from a point 4 to 5 mm nasal to the punctum (care is taken not to extend the incision into the caruncle) to a point 4 to 5 mm temporal to the punctum. The conjunctival incision edges are overlapped, rotating the punctum posteriorly. When the rotation is sufficient to replace the inferior punctum into the lacrimal lake, the inferior edge of the palpebral conjunctiva is resected where it overlaps the superior wound edge. The incisions and simultaneous hemostasis can be conveniently performed using a CO_2 laser or a fine-wire radiosurgery electrode (Ellman International, Hewlett, NY). Additional cautery and/or vaporization of the submucosa will augment fibrosis and posterior rotation of the punctum. This technique is most easily performed with complete hemostasis using a radiosurgical electrode (blended cutting-hemostasis waveform) or a 0.2-mm CO_2 laser handpiece. The wound is closed with buried interrupted 6-0 plain sutures. A chalazion clamp may be used to stabilize the lid margin and provide adequate countertraction and hemostasis, but it must be released when the height of the palpebral conjunctival resection is determined, and care must be taken not to crush the inferior canaliculus with the clamp.

If punctal eversion is marked, unrelieved with massage, and unassociated with lower lid margin horizontal laxity, and if there is nasal lid margin retraction on upward gaze, a retroauricular free-skin graft and lysis of subcutaneous adhesions will be necessary to release the punctum from the anterior lamellar cicatrix. An elliptical free-skin graft can be placed segmentally into the lower lid just anterior to the punctum, if there is no evidence of other cicatricial lid margin distortion.

Ectropion (Anterior Lamellar Shortening)

In the era of lower lid cutaneous resections, excessive skin resections everted the lower lid margin (Fig. 6). Patients with heavy jowls and ptotic, redundant midfacial soft tissues were predisposed to lower lid ectropion, even without aggressive skin resection. It is conceivable that aggressive lower lid laser resurfacing applied to the pretarsal skin of a lid with lid margin laxity could cause eversion of the lower lid margin, as well as lower lid margin retraction.

Mild lid margin eversion can be corrected with upward massage for at least 5 minutes four times daily. The massage therapy should be continued for as long as improve-

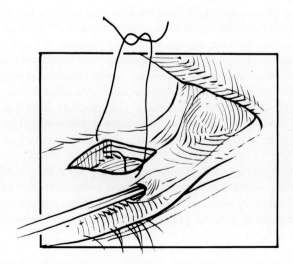

FIG. 5. Mild inferior punctal eversion is remedied with a retropunctal palpebral conjunctival resection. The canaliculus is retracted and identified with a Bowman probe.

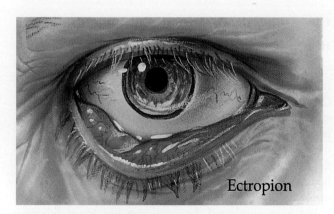

FIG. 6. The risk of lower lid ectropion has been greatly diminished since the advent and practice of lower lid transconjunctival blepharoplasty.

ment is noted. Increased lower lid resilience and scar stretching and softening may result in an improvement even 6 months after the procedure. However, persistent lower lid margin malposition after 6 to 8 weeks of massage will most likely need surgical repair.

Mild lower lid margin displacement may be corrected with lateral canthal tendon plication. With the patient sitting in an upright position, the surgeon can approximate lateral canthal tightening with his or her finger and can visualize the effect on the lid margin position.

Unimproving or long-standing lower lid ectropion following transcutaneous blepharoplasty should be managed as a cicatricial ectropion. A series of postoperative photographs will help the surgeon make the decision about the degree of improvement and preclude subjective visual bias. Free-skin grafting is the definitive technique for surgical correction. A 4-0 black silk suture is placed in and out of the gray line in the midline of the lower lid and clamped to the sterile drapes superiorly, stabilizing the lid margin and keeping the lower lid on maximum stretch. A subciliary incision is made from the inferior punctum to the lateral canthal angle. Any adhesions between skin and orbicularis muscle as far inferiorly as the inferior orbital rim are lysed. After release of these adhesions, the gap between the superiorly retracted subciliary incision and inferior wound edge is the height of the anterior lamellar deficit that must be corrected (Fig. 7). The shape and dimensions of the elliptical defect are noted, or a template is made of a suture wrapper.

A full-thickness retroauricular skin graft is demarcated and injected subcutaneously with a solution of lidocaine 2% with 1:200,000 epinephrine. Although some mild contraction of the graft can be expected, if too large a skin graft is used, the redundant fold will not please the cosmetic blepharoplasty patient. A slight overcorrection, however, is preferable to a slight undercorrection. The graft is fixated in the host bed with four cardial sutures of 6-0 black silk (two superior and two inferior). Care is taken not to place them through the tapered edges of the graft, where sloughing is possible. A running, locking 6-0 nylon suture anastomoses the host–donor junction. After removal of the protective lens, the 4-0 black silk traction suture is sutured to the thick skin above the brow, keeping the lower lid on maximum stretch and immobilizing the graft. Several stab incisions are made in the graft for possible hematoma drainage. A combination steroid–antibiotic ophthalmic ointment is applied to the graft. A modified pressure dressing of rolled Telfa and two eye patches further immobilizes the graft and prevents hematoma formation between the host bed and the graft. The patch is removed on the second postoperative day. The traction and graft sutures are removed after 5 days. The patient should not expect complete color blending of the graft with the host until 3 to 6 months after surgery.

In cases of long-standing cicatricial ectropion, there is a gradual elongation of the lid margin that will require lateral

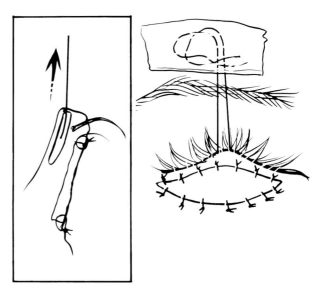

FIG. 7. The lower lid is stabilized with a traction suture fixated above the brow. A retroauricular graft is used to correct the anterior lamellar defect.

canthal tightening, as well as free-skin grafting of the anterior lamella. The lower lid is maximally stretched with a 4-0 black silk traction suture clamped to the sterile drapes superiorly. If there is a subciliary scar, it is incised; the skin flap is undermined as far inferiorly as the inferior orbital rim. The subcutaneous cicatrix is lysed and excised. The traction suture is released.

A lateral canthal tendon plication will correct mild and moderate lower lid margin laxity. In more severe cases, a lateral wedge resection of the lower lid margin with a lateral tarsal strip suspension will be necessary.

An inverted, pentagonal resection of the lower lid is performed temporally. To accurately assess lid apposition to the globe, the opaque corneal protector should be removed before the pentagonal resection is performed. The width of the inverted, pentagonal resection is determined by overlapping the severed ends of the lid margin until the lid margin is in tight apposition to the globe. The nasal segment of the lid margin is notched with Wesscott scissors at the point where it overlaps the temporal lid margin. A strip of tarsus is spared.

After the lid resection is completed, the corneal protector may be replaced. The lateral tarsal strip is anchored to the periosteum of the internal aspect of the lateral orbital rim. The lid margin is reapproximated with interrupted 6-0 black silk sutures placed in the lash line, the meibomian orifices, and the gray line. The suture ends are left 10 mm long.

The tarsus and conjunctiva are closed in one layer with interrupted 5-0 chromic sutures. The traction suture is again fixated superiorly. A template for the skin graft may be fashioned. The retroauricular free-skin graft is sutured into the host bed. The long ends of the lid margin sutures are anchored to the superior graft–host wound edge to avoid postoperative corneal epithelial erosion. The corneal protector is removed. The traction suture is sutured to the thick skin above the brow. The retroauricular donor site is closed with 4-0 chromic vertical mattress sutures. A combination steroid–antibiotic ophthalmic ointment is applied to the wounds. A modified pressure dressing of rolled Telfa and two eye patches is applied to the graft site. Rolled Telfa is applied to the retroauricular donor site.

Ectropion (with Horizontal Laxity)

Preoperative horizontal laxity of the lower lid margin or canthal tendons may cause a postblepharoplasty lid margin eversion if a cutaneous approach is used or pretarsal resurfacing is performed. If horizontal laxity is present preoperatively, a lid margin tightening or a lateral canthal supportive procedure must be performed during the initial procedure. Lower lid horizontal laxity can be determined preoperatively by distracting the lid at least 6 to 8 mm from the globe. Nasal traction displacing the lateral canthal angle more than 2 mm toward the temporal limbus denotes lateral canthal tendon laxity. Correction within the early postoperative period may be accomplished with a lateral canthal tendon plication. Thereafter, long-standing cutaneous cicatrization may necessitate a lateral tarsal strip suspension of the lateral canthus with recession of the lower lid retractors and a free retroauricular skin graft.

Lower Lid Retraction with Inferior Scleral Show

Postoperative widening of the palpebral aperture with increased inferior scleral show is not a desired result (Fig. 8A,B). In addition to the change in shape of the patient's eyes, lagophthalmos also may result. Lower lid retraction may occur without ectropion. It is accentuated on upward gaze and may be accompanied by anterior displacement of the lid margin on upward gaze. It may be caused by excessive skin resection or cutaneous cicatrization without skin resection. Lower lid retraction may be secondary to aggressive horizontal lid shortening in a patient with prominent eyes, shallow orbits, undiagnosed thyroid ophthalmopathy, and preexisting inferior scleral show.

The cause of lower lid retraction may not be evident before corrective procedures are attempted. On upward gaze, if the lower lid skin is tight and maximally stretched, excessive skin resection or laser resurfacing may be the cause, and free-skin grafting is the cure. If a horizontal shortening had been performed and there appears to be adequate lower lid skin, but the horizontal palpebral aperture is slightly narrowed and a review of the preoperative photographs reveals a preexisting inferior scleral show, the lower lid probably has been tightened onto the convex inferior surface of the globe. Thus, in the upright position, the lower lid margin cannot be maintained and slides farther inferiorly on the globe. Correction of this complication is not always satisfactory. It requires recession of the lower lid retractors, with or without grafting of hard palate, mucous membrane, or donor sclera, and superiorly directed support from a lateral canthal plication or a lateral tarsal strip (Fig. 9). Preoperative inferior scleral show is a clear indication for the transconjunctival approach to lower lid fat resections.

Rounding of Lateral Canthal Angle

Any alteration or distortion of the acute lateral canthal angle is quite apparent and requires correction (Table 1). Excessive lower lid skin or skin–muscle resections, particularly when extended to the lateral orbital rim, may blunt the lateral canthal angle or cause an inferior displacement of the angle. Lateral tarsal strips that have dehisced or torn through their periorbital attachments may also round the lateral canthal angle. Aggressive laser resurfacing of the lower lids can result in lower lid retraction, narrowing of the horizontal palpebral aperture, and rounding of the lateral canthal angle.

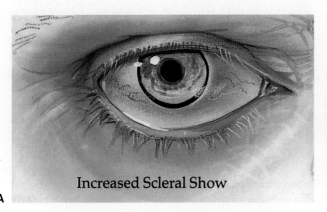
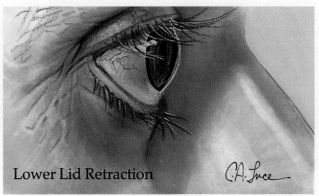

Increased Scleral Show

Lower Lid Retraction

A

B

FIG. 8. A,B: Transconjunctival blepharoplasty has minimized the risk of lower lid retraction and the accentuation of preexisting inferior scleral show.

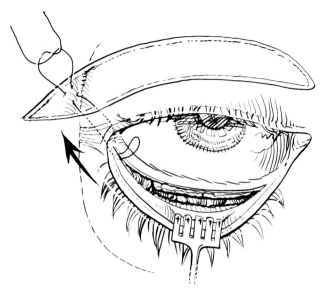

FIG. 9. Lower lid retraction may be corrected in most patients by recessing the lower lid retractors transconjunctivally and suspending the lateral canthus.

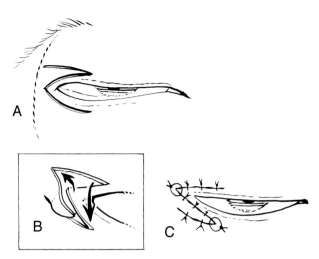

FIG. 10. A: A lateral transposition flap of upper lid skin can be used to correct deficiencies of temporal lower lid skin, elevate the lateral canthal angle, and correct rounding. **B:** The flaps are mobilized, undermined, and transposed. **C:** The lids and canthus should be in place when the flaps are sutured.

Cicatricial deformities of short duration without associated laxity of the lid margin or lateral canthal tendon can be effectively corrected with a free-skin graft. Deformities of long duration with secondary lateral canthal tendon and lid margin laxity may need a free-skin graft with a lateral tarsal strip and recession of lower lid retractors. A mild lateral ectropion with rounded lateral canthal angle and a minimal cicatricial component will respond nicely to a lateral tarsal strip without a free-skin graft. Inferior displacements of the lateral canthal angle may be remedied with a temporal transposition flap from the upper lid to the lower lid (Fig. 10A), release of subcutaneous cicatrix, recession of lower lid retractors, and lateral canthal plication. A subciliary incision of the lower lid is demarcated along the displaced temporal lower lid margin as far as the lateral orbital rim. A corresponding supraciliary incision of the upper lid joins the inferior incision at the lateral orbital rim to form an acute angle. The height of the temporally based triangular transposition flap is determined by the amount of lateral canthal angle elevation desired. The superior edge

of this flap is drawn as a horizontal line at the desired level of canthal angle repositioning and joins the supraciliary incision, forming the apex of the triangular flap. The demarcated incisions are incised. Extensive undermining is performed to permit adequate mobilization of the canthal angle, lower lid margin, and transposition flap, as well as sufficient release of the cicatricial bed inferiorly (Fig. 10B). The flap is transposed and sutured into place with interrupted 6-0 nylon sutures (Fig. 10C).

Lymphedema

Postblepharoplasty lymphedema is a rare but frustrating sequel to cosmetic surgery. The transconjunctival approach has virtually eliminated this complication. Avoiding placement of the lateral extension of a subciliary incision closer than 4 mm to the lateral palpebral raphe and not joining the lower lid incision to the upper lid incision may eliminate lymphedema. It may take up to 1 year for the boggy, sometimes erythematous appearance of the lower lid to subside. Lymphatic drainage massage may also provide a transient decrease in the lymphedema, and repeated treatments may provide longer lasting improvement.

Extraocular Muscle Imbalance

The inferior oblique tendon courses between the nasal and middle inferior fat pockets. Aggressive fat resection without regard for this structure may result in damage to the tendon, with resultant weakening of inferior oblique function. Aggressive cauterization of the fat pad stumps in this region may result in fibrosis of the tendon. Awareness

TABLE 1. *Correction of rounding of lateral canthal angle*

1. Lateral canthal plication
2. Lateral canthal plication plus recession of lower lid retractors
3. Lateral canthal plication, lower lid retractor recession, lateral transposition flap
4. Lateral canthal plication and retractor recession plus free-skin graft
5. Lateral tarsal strip suspension and recession of lower lid retractors plus free-skin graft

of the location of the inferior oblique tendon can eliminate these complications.

Recognition of the inferior oblique is particularly relevant when a transconjunctival blepharoplasty is performed. It is much more easily exposed and identified when this approach is utilized.

Inferior Sulcus Asymmetry

The transconjunctival approach and laser vaporization of prolapsing fat allow easier assessment of the lower lid contour and greater accuracy of liposculpting. However, excessive fat resection may yield an inappropriately deep concavity of the inferior sulcus. This may be difficult to correct, but the implantation of free fat pearls or transplantation of fat pedicle flaps has been used with some success. Hyaluronic acid gel injections have also yielded long-term improvement.

Residual fat will require transconjunctival exploration (Fig. 11). CO_2 laser vaporization of residual pockets can be performed with great accuracy.

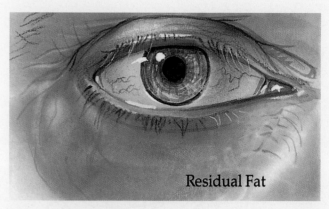

Residual Fat

FIG. 11. Residual lower lid fat can be accurately vaporized with a CO_2 laser via a transconjunctival approach.

CHAPTER 11

Laser Eyelid Rejuvenation

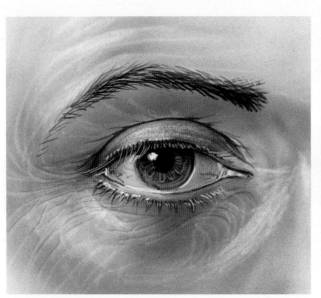
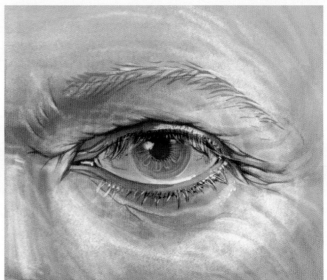

Clearly, the carbon dioxide (CO_2) laser not only facilitates the performance of cosmetic blepharoplasty but also enhances the potential result. An essentially bloodless incisional technique combined with eyelid resurfacing (utilizing a computer pattern generator and supplemented with application of an erbium:yttrium-aluminum-garnet [Er:YAG] laser) can yield a quality of result not previously attainable. There is no doubt, however, that there is a learning curve necessary to master this technique and fully comprehend the new aesthetic of laser blepharoplasty.

The first lesson to be learned is the no-touch technique for incision and soft tissue dissection. This is simplified by the use of the aiming bar that fits onto the tip of the 0.2-mm cutting handpiece. CO_2 laser incisions require that the beam be exactly in focus for effective cutting. If the instrument is held too close or too far from the tissue, the beam will be defocused, and there will be more lateral heat spread and less cutting. When a blood vessel is encountered, the beam can be purposefully defocused to obliterate it; this will be necessary for vessels larger than 0.5 mm in diameter (Fig. 1B). When incising and dissecting, the surgeon must move quickly. Applying laser energy too long in one spot will generate too much lateral heat spread and char the tissue (Fig. 1A). This can also be minimized by moistening the wound edges. The laser surgeon must also learn to reidentify anatomic landmarks in a completely hemostatic environment. The tissue planes will have a new color and texture.

Almost all patients can be candidates for incisional and resurfacing laser eyelid rejuvenation. With appropriate preparation and postoperative care, even patients with darker skin types can be treated with excellent results. We have had a large and rewarding experience treating Asian and black-skinned patients (Fig. 2A,B).

The laser surgeon must respect the power and realize the potential of the laser. Because of its ease of use, especially when resurfacing, the surgeon must resist excessive application of laser energy. The lower lid margin may be particularly vulnerable to lower lid margin displacement and should be treated with caution. Direct vaporization of preaponeurotic and suborbicularis brow fat can effectively recontour the areas to which it is directed.

After repair of aponeurotic disinsertion, light, defocused application of the CO_2 laser to the aponeurosis can cause elevation of the lid margin. This maneuver, when understood and utilized with care, can yield superb results. If the surgeon is unaware of this effect, however, upper lid retraction may be the sequel.

UPPER LID INCISIONAL TECHNIQUE

Handpiece: 0.2 mm.
Laser settings:
—For skin and conjunctiva: 5 mJ, 5 W (UltraPulse) (Coherent Medical, Palo Alto, CA).
—For orbicularis and fat: 5 to 8 mJ, 5 W (UltraPulse or continuous wave).

Myocutaneous Incisions and Resections

A metallic, nonreflective corneal protector is placed on the cornea, or a nonreflective metal lid plate is held behind the lid to protect the globe. Subcutaneous infiltration of anesthetic is given using a 30-gauge needle. A bolus of anesthetic solution is massaged across the lid, avoiding excess puncture sites and the possibility of a hematoma (Fig. 3).

The previously demarcated skin incisions are slightly moistened and incised. Care is taken to move the handpiece quickly and to keep the beam focused to avoid charring the wound edges. To minimize lateral heat spread, the UltraPulse modality is preferred over the continuous wave made when incising the skin and conjunctiva.

A second pass incises the orbicularis muscle. The lateral edge of the myocutaneous flap is grasped, and the flap is then undermined in the nasal direction with transverse passes of the laser (see Fig. 1A).

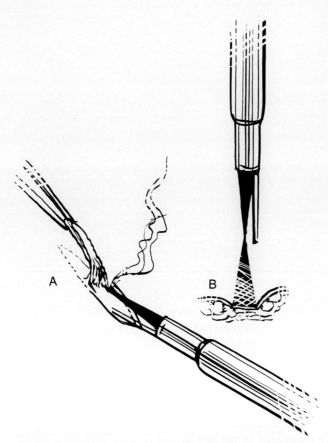

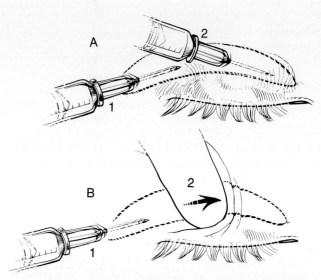

FIG. 1. A: The CO_2 laser is a superb cutting tool, when used for incisions. The surgeon must move quickly to avoid lateral heat spread. **B:** The CO_2 laser will obliterate blood vessels and shrink fat when the beam is defocused by moving it away from the tissue.

FIG. 3. To minimize bruising from multiple subcutaneous infiltrations, **(A)** a bolus of anesthetic solution is injected laterally (*1*) and massaged across the upper lid (*2*) **(B)**.

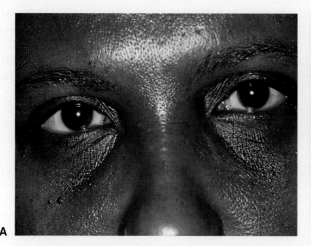

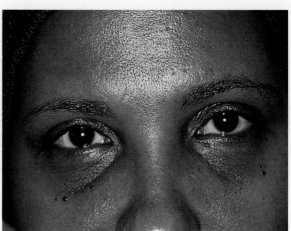

FIG. 2. A: This young black-skinned woman had lower lid hyperpigmentation and poor skin texture.
B: She responded well to topical bleaching agents, peels, and CO_2 laser lower lid resurfacing.

Fat Resection and Direct Vaporization

Gentle pressure on the globe causes the prolapsing fat to bulge against the septum. As the nasal aspect of the septum is incised, the fat pours through the septal opening. It is grasped, folded over a moistened cotton-tipped applicator, and then incised. Residual fat is vaporized directly. For enhanced cutting or increased hemostatic capability, the power may be increased to 8 mJ and the mode changed to continuous wave.

The septal incision is extended laterally, exposing the central fat pocket. It is incised over a cotton-tipped applicator, and any residual fat is vaporized directly.

Suborbicularis Fat Pocket (Brow Fat Pocket) Resection

The upper lid myocutaneous flap is extended superiorly 5 to 10 mm beyond the superior orbital rim. The fat lying in this suborbicularis muscle plane, anterior to the periosteum, is resected. This pocket tends to be very vascular and bleeding can be minimized by keeping the base of the resection at the level of the periosteum and by defocusing the laser to obliterate vessels as they are encountered. It is convenient to begin the dissection laterally and to complete the resection just before the supraorbital bundle is reached; this will avoid supraorbital paresthesia and bleeding. After this resection is completed, any residual fat or adherent orbicularis muscle can be vaporized directly, and internal brow suspension can be performed (Fig. 4).

LOWER LID INCISIONAL TECHNIQUES (TRANSCONJUNCTIVAL)

Handpiece: 0.2 mm.
Laser settings:
   —For conjunctiva: 5 mJ, 5 W (UltraPulse).
   —For fat: 5 to 8 mJ (UltraPulse or continuous wave).

Since the demonstration of the effectiveness of resurfacing, there is rarely an indication for lower lid skin resection. We feel that there is never an indication for a subciliary incision or a myocutaneous flap. In patients with an extreme excess of lower lid skin, a conservative pinch technique in the lower lid crease may be combined with lower lid resurfacing.

A metallic nonreflective corneal protector is put into place to protect the globe. An inferior transcutaneous peribulbar block may be supplemented with an inferior fornix intraorbital regional block.

The conjunctiva is incised midway between the inferior tarsal margin and the inferior fornix. As gentle pressure is applied to the globe, the prolapsing fat causes a bulge in the inferior palpebral conjunctiva. Incision the conjunctiva over the bulge will facilitate localization of the prolapsed fat. A second pass is necessary to incise the lower lid retractors centrally, allowing the fat to prolapse. The central fat pocket is incised over a moistened cotton-tipped applicator, and residual fat is directly vaporized (Fig. 5). The conjunctival and lower lid retractor incisions are extended laterally and nasally, stopping just lateral to the caruncle. The inferior oblique is identified between the central and nasal fat pockets. The nasal fat pocket is resected and vaporized. The lateral fat pocket is resected and vaporized. Gentle pressure is applied to the globe and the inferior sulcus is palpated for residual contour irregularities. Additional lipocontouring by direct vaporization and resection can then be performed. When the contour is acceptable, the lower lid margin is pulled superiorly and the anterior lamella smoothed with the surgeon's finger; this maneuver will release any potential adhesions of the lower lid retractors.

UPPER LID RESURFACING TECHNIQUES

In patients with mild lid fold redundancy and no fatty prolapse, upper lid resurfacing without myocutaneous re-

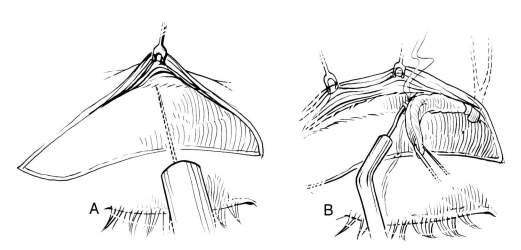

FIG. 4. After a myocutaneous flap is developed superiorly, exposing the superior orbital rim, the suborbicularis brow fat pocket is resected and/or directly vaporized.

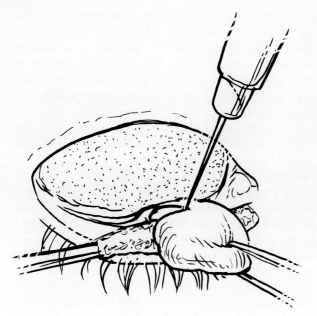

FIG. 5. Via the transconjunctival approach, the retractors are incised, and the fat prolapses and is then resected over a moistened cotton-tipped applicator. Any residual fat is vaporized directly.

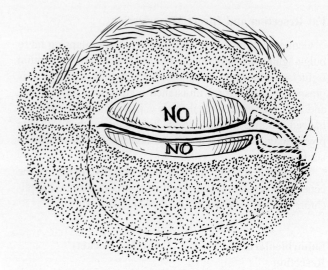

FIG. 7. Unless there is exceptional wrinkling of the pretarsal area, this area is usually avoided when the eyelids are resurfaced with a CO_2 laser. Pretarsal resurfacing with the Er: YAG laser can be accomplished with less potential for lid margin displacement.

section can effectively recontour the upper lid, while improving the skin texture (Fig. 6A,B).

Unless the pretarsal skin is exceptionally wrinkled, this area is not treated. The area to be resurfaced extends from the upper lid crease to the brow, is extended as far laterally as the most lateral extent of the crow's-feet or laugh line deformity, and can be extended as far medially as the bridge of the nose (Fig. 7). The quality of skin, the amount of rhytids, and the extent of the lid fold overlap will determine the area to be resurfaced and the potency of the treatment.

Care should be taken not to singe the eyebrow hair. The brow may be protected with a metallic nonreflective shield or by application of a sterile lubricant. A small square pattern is used (pattern 3, size 4) with a density of 5 or 6 (Fig. 8). One, two, or three passes are used, with the power settings on the initial pass ranging from 200 to 300 mJ. Power settings on the second or third pass range from 150 to 250 mJ; 60 W are used on all passes.

In patients with fine upper lid rhytidosis, when only minimal skin contraction is required, the Er:YAG laser is useful (5-mm spot, 2 J, two to three passes).

The art of resurfacing involves a comprehensive and effective utilization of the variables. This is not only a function of the power (millijoules) but also a function of the

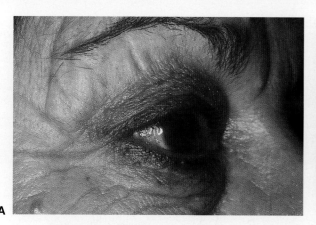

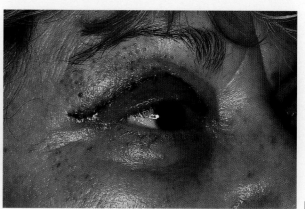

FIG. 6. A: This 58-year-old woman had marked eyelid rhytidosis. This degree of eyelid skin texture abnormality is not amenable to incisional techniques alone. **B:** Two days following upper and lower lid transconjunctival blepharoplasties with periocular CO_2 laser resurfacing, she shows a striking improvement in eyelid contour and texture.

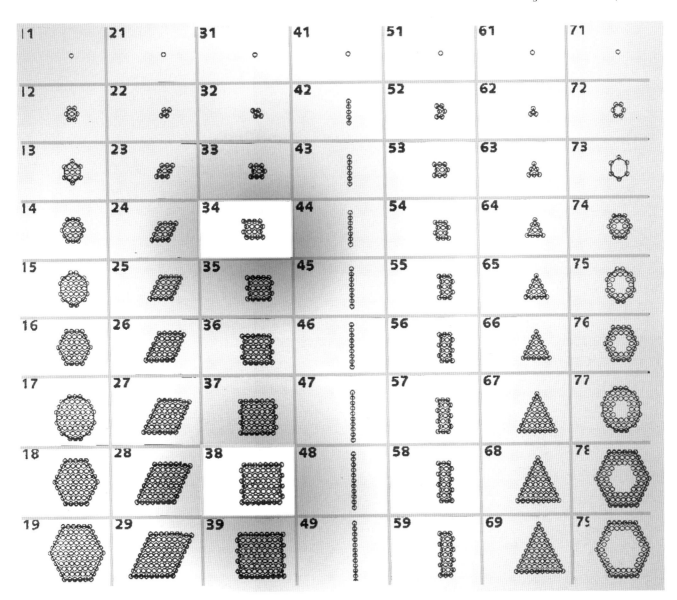

FIG. 8. Pattern 3, size 4, density 5 or 6 is used for resurfacing the eyelids, with power ranging from 150 to 300 mJ, depending on the desired degree of rhytid ablation or tissue tightening.

area treated in one application (pattern and pattern size), the speed of the application (watts), and the density of the application. We like to use the UltraPulse CO_2 laser because it allows us to use these variables and gives us a great margin of safety.

LOWER LID RESURFACING TECHNIQUES

The combination of lower lid transconjunctival lipocontouring and lower lid resurfacing achieves a better result with fewer complications than the transcutaneous approach to the lower lids (Fig. 9A–D). In addition, there is a dramatic decrease in the incidence of postoperative lower lid retraction following the transconjunctival approach with lower lid resurfacing.

There are several areas that deserve special attention when lower lid resurfacing is considered. If there is any horizontal laxity of the lower lid margin or lateral canthal tendon, the lateral canthal tendon should be plicated before resurfacing of the lower lid skin. (Tables 1 and 2). When the pretarsal skin is resurfaced, lower density and power

TABLE 1. *Lower lid resurfacing: points of caution*

Correct lid margin laxity
Approach pretarsal area cautiously
Avoid prepunctal area
Avoid overtreatment

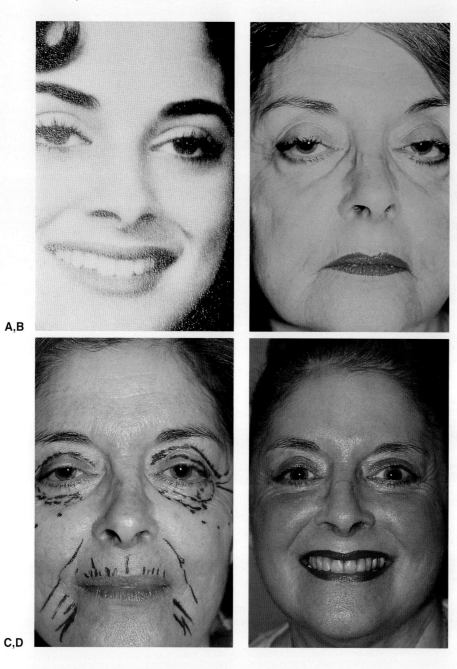

A,B

C,D

FIG. 9. A: An old photograph of this patient is used to determine the proposed lid and facial contours. **B:** Preoperatively, she had bilateral upper lid ptosis, lower lid retraction, and multiple areas of facial sagging. **C:** Levator aponeurotic advancements, upper lid myocutaneous resections, and lipocontouring, were planned, as well as transconjunctival lipocontouring and recession of lower lid retractors, lateral canthoplasties, and full-face laser resurfacing. **D:** Postoperatively, her lid levels and contours are improved. Elevating the lower lid margins transconjunctivally and combining the technique with resurfacing avoided further displacement of the lower lid margin.

should be used, and resurfacing should not proceed nasal to the inferior punctum. Lower lid pretarsal resurfacing is only indicated for extreme rhytidosis, marked dermal patina, or prominent pretarsal orbicularis hypertrophy.

The parameters for lower lid CO_2 resurfacing differ slightly from those of the upper lid. The power and density of the first pass should vary with the area treated: The pre-

TABLE 2. *Rejuvenating a lax lower lid*

Lateral canthal plication
Resurface lateral canthus first
Avoid pretarsal resurfacing

tarsal area is treated the least; the entire premalar area is treated more heavily (Table 3). For fine lower lid rhytidosis, the Er:YAG laser can be used. Because there is less skin contraction with its use, the pretarsal skin may be treated with less chance of secondary lower lid margin malposition.

ALTERNATIVE EYELID REJUVENATION TECHNIQUES: ER:YAG LASER

The Er:YAG laser (2,940 mμ wavelength) can be of benefit to patients with fine periocular rhytids. Using a 5-mm spot with 1 to 2 J and a slow rate (4 pulses per second), it can be used without intravenous sedation or subcutaneous

TABLE 3. *Lower lid resurfacing parameters (mJ)*

Pass	Pretarsal	Preseptal	Premalar
First	150–200	200–300	250–300
Second	150	200–300	250–300
Third	—	150–200	250–300

injection. After application of topical anesthetic paste for 20 to 40 minutes, each rhytid can be visualized and its response to laser treatment observed.

Following botulinum toxin type A purified neurotoxin complex (Botox) injections, use of an Er:YAG laser in the crow's-feet area can be effective for fine residual rhytidosis.

A 5-mm spot with 1 J may require four to five passes. A 5-mm spot with 2 J may require two to three passes.

The immediate postoperative course is different from that of patients having CO_2 laser resurfacing. There may be some oozing of blood. Because of less thermal effect, however, the recovery time will be shorter.

CHAPTER 12

Laser Facial Rejuvenation

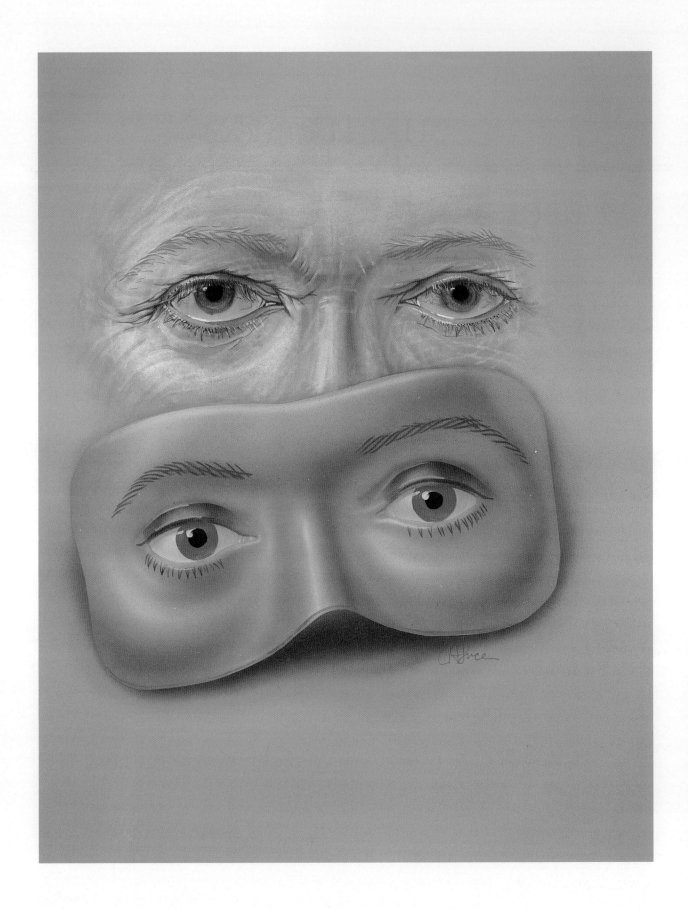

The introduction of facial rejuvenation resurfacing techniques with the carbon dioxide (CO_2) laser has significantly expanded the therapeutic options for patients (Fig. 1A–F). To master this procedure, the cosmetic surgeon must understand the principles of how the laser functions and the aesthetics of its application, must spend time with a preceptor or preceptors and grasp the insights gained by their experience, and then proceed cautiously. CO_2 laser resurfacing is technically simple; its use is not confined to any one medical discipline or specialty. The difficulty is in mastering the aesthetics of the techniques. This is what requires experience and training. This is a tool that can be used potentially for great benefit, but its misuse can create complications just as any surgical procedure can (Fig. 2).

GENERAL PRINCIPLES OF LASER FACIAL REJUVENATION

CO_2 facial rejuvenation can be performed in an outpatient setting with intravenous sedation, regional blocks, and local infiltration. The nerve blocks that work with a high degree of success are supraorbital, supratrochlear, infratrochlear, infraorbital, zygomaticofacial, facial, and mental; these are supplemented with local infiltration (Fig. 3).

The basic principles are as follows: The first pass deepithelializes the skin; the second and third passes level surface irregularities and tighten the dermis. More elevated lesions require repeated applications using a single spot. These lesions are vaporized before the generalized resurfacing is performed. We rarely use more than three passes during a session, except in patients with rhinophyma and in some acne patients. More than three passes reduces the margin of safety and risks damage to the deep reticular dermis. Surgeon and patient cannot lose if the dictum "you can always do more" is followed. Using color changes in the skin between laser applications as a guide to which dermal layer has received laser energy (stopping when a

chamois color is achieved) and as an indication of a therapeutic end point is not always reliable.

The periocular fascial structures are the most delicate and must be treated in a manner different from the rest of the face. These parameters have been discussed separately in chapter 11.

The intensity of the treatment will be modified by the thickness of the skin and the degree of actinic damage. We have found that the more severe the actinic changes are, the more dramatic the result is. Rhytid ablation will be more prominent, and the lifting effect more significant (Figs. 4A–F, 5A,B). Patients who have previously undergone rhytidectomy but have residual rhytidosis respond well to postrhytidectomy laser resurfacing performed at least 3 to 6 months following the initial procedure. In patients with translucent, thin skin, we rarely apply more than two passes with the UltraPulse CO_2 laser (Coherent, Palo Alto, CA) (Tables 1 and 2).

The resurfacing parameters will differ with the instrument used. Pulsed CO_2 laser and scanning CO_2 laser applications will differ in the power used and the number of passes utilized. As an example, one pass of the Silk Touch (Sharplan Lasers, Allendale, NJ) may be equal to two passes with the UltraPulse (Coherent Medical, Palo Alto, Calif).

Full-face CO_2 laser resurfacing is conveniently and effectively performed concomitantly with upper and lower lid blepharoplasty, lateral canthoplasty, levator aponeurotic advancement, and internal brow suspension (Fig. 6A,B). Botulinum toxin type A purified neurotoxin complex (Botox) injection 1 week before the resurfacing or at the conclusion of the resurfacing will enhance cosmetic improvement for the glabellar, crow's-feet, and forehead regions (dynamic rhytids).

Full-face laser resurfacing includes applications to every area of the face, including the upper and lower lids, nose, and lips (Fig. 7). The exposed lip mucosa can be resurfaced

(text continues on page 136)

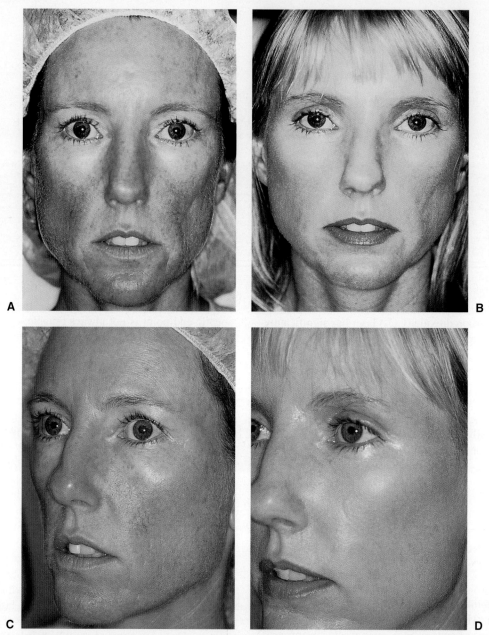

FIG. 1. A: This 33-year-old woman had severe actinic damage and moderate acne scarring. **B:** Her appearance shows striking improvement 2 weeks following upper lid sculpting, lower lid transconjunctival lipocontouring, and full-face CO_2 laser resurfacing (face: pattern 3, size 8, density 6, 300 mJ, two passes, third pass: acne scared areas only; eyes: pattern 3, size 4, density 6, 250 mJ first pass, 200 mJ second pass). She is wearing makeup. **C,D:** Oblique views.

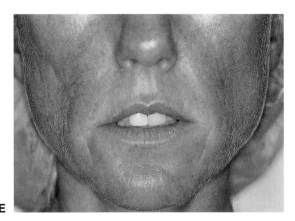 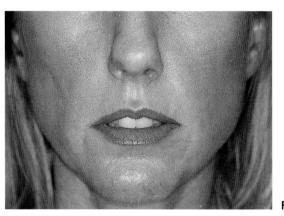

FIG. 1. *Continued.* **E,F:** Lower facial views.

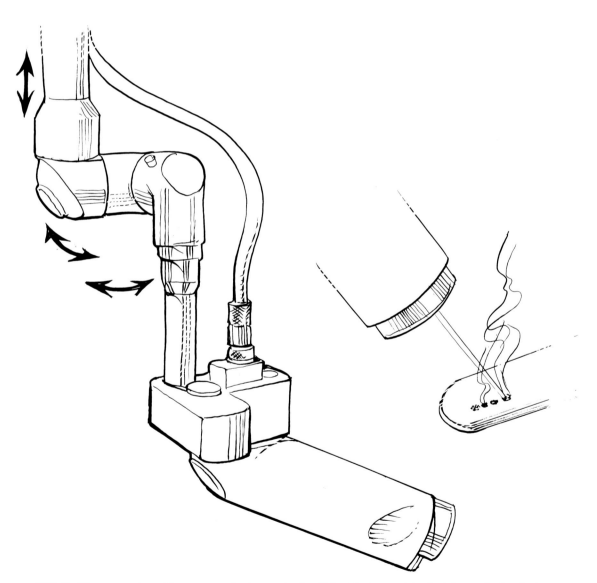

FIG. 2. The computer pattern generator is a potent, efficient instrument for facial resurfacing that can be used with a great margin of safety.

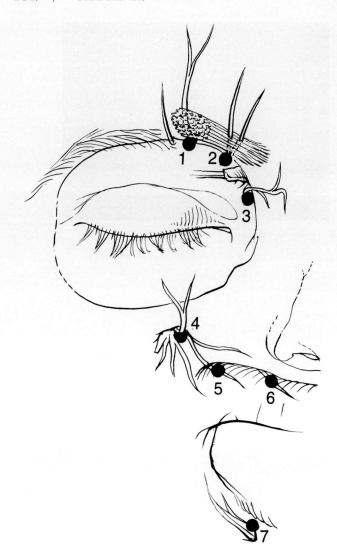

FIG. 3. The effective use of regional nerve blocks greatly facilitates facial resurfacing; the most frequently used are supraorbital (*1*), supratrochlear (*2*), infratrochlear (*3*), infraorbital (*4*), zygomaticofacial (*5*), nasal (*6*), and mental (*7*). The last two blocks are given intraorally.

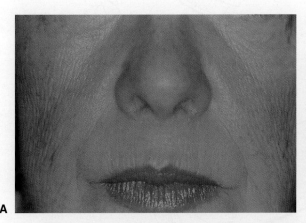

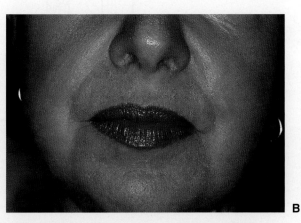

FIG. 4. A: This 56-year-old woman had moderate to marked facial actinic changes and had multiple facial basal cell carcinomas removed. **B:** Three weeks following full-face CO_2 laser resurfacing (pattern 3, size 8, density 6, 300 mJ, three passes; eyelids: pattern 3, size 4, density 5, 200 mJ first pass, 150 mJ second pass), she has a dramatic reduction in her facial rhytids and a dramatic improvement in her facial contour. Moderate facial erythema persists.

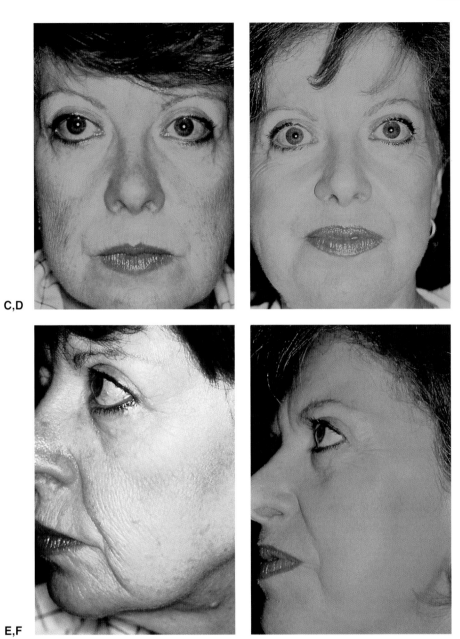

C,D

E,F

FIG. 4 *Continued.* By the tenth post-treatment week, her facial skin color reapproximates that of her youth **(C,D)**, and her facial contour shows further improvement **(E,F)**.

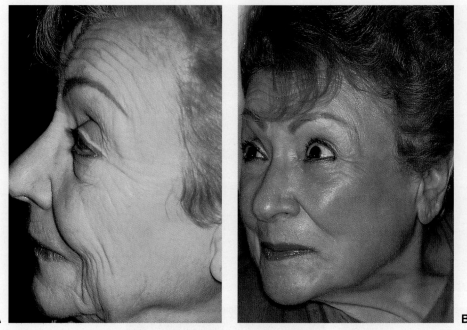

FIG. 5. A: This 82-year-old woman had marked facial rhytidosis and facial laxity. **B:** Six weeks following full-face resurfacing (pattern 3, size 8, density 6, 300 mJ first pass, 250 mJ second and third passes), levator aponeurotic repair, and transconjunctival lipocontouring she shows a marked decrease in her facial rhytidosis and a prominent tightening of her facial contours.

TABLE 1. *Full-face CO_2 laser resurfacing parameters: thick skin*

Facial rhytidosis	Passes (no.)	First pass (mJ)	Second pass (mJ)	Third pass (mJ)	Improvement (%)
1+	2	250	200	—	60
2+	2	250	250	—	70
3+	2	300	300	—	80
4+	3	300	300	300	85

TABLE 2. *Full-face CO_2 laser resurfacing parameters: thin skin*

Facial rhytidosis	Passes (no.)	First pass (mJ)	Second pass (mJ)	Third pass (mJ)	Improvement (%)
1+	1	250	—	—	50
2+	2	250	200	—	60
3+	2	250	250	—	70
4+	2	300	250	—	75

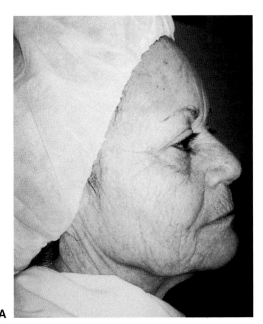
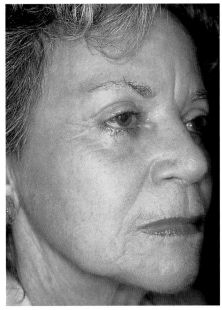

FIG. 6. A: This 75-year-old woman had severe actinic changes of her facial skin. **B:** Six weeks following upper lid myocutaneous resections and lipocontouring, lower lid transconjunctival lipocontouring, and full-face resurfacing (face: pattern 3, size 8, density 6, 300 mJ, three passes; eyelids: pattern 3, size 4, density 6, 250 mJ, two passes, she shows a marked improvement of her eyelid and facial contours and texture.

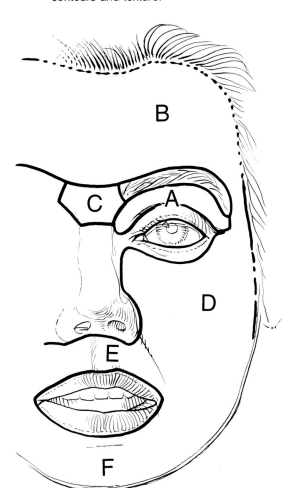

FIG. 7. Customized plan for facial resurfacing. Eyelids: (a) pretarsal: CO_2 laser: 0–2 passes, 150–200 mJ; Er:YAG laser: 1–3 passes, 2 J, 5-mm spot; (b) preseptal: CO_2 laser: 1–3 passes 150–250 mJ; Er:YAG laser: 3–5 passes, 2 J, 5-mm spot. Forehead: (pretreated with Botox): CO_2 laser: 1–3 passes, 250–300 mJ; Er:YAG laser: 1 pass following CO_2 passes, 2 J, 5-mm spot. Cheeks, chin: CO_2 laser: 1–3 passes, 250–300 mJ; Er:YAG laser: 1–4 passes following CO_2 passes, 2 J, 5-mm spot. Upper lip: CO_2 laser: 1–3 passes, 250–300 mJ; Er:YAG laser: 1–4 passes following CO_2 passes, 2 J, 5-mm spot.

if actinic cheilitis are evident. The earlobes also may be resurfaced if they show actinic changes or are stretched. During full-face resurfacing, we treat larger areas with each pass of the laser. With the computer pattern generator (CPG) (Fig. 8), we use pattern 3, size 8 or 9 with a density of 6. With the Silk Touch we use 9- or 12-mm spot sizes. The resurfacing is feathered into the scalp and feathered 2 cm beyond the turning of the mandible; this will make any transitional demarcation in skin texture less apparent. Pigmentary demarcation lines are transient.

Feathering is performed either by tilting the collimated CPG beam and causing oblique applications of the laser or by decreasing the power (millijoules) of the machine. Non-collimated lasers can be defocused (pulling the handpiece away from the tissue) to feather. TCA (Trichloro acetic acid) peels can also be used in these transitional areas.

RULES OF THUMB

The heavier the treatment is, the more intense the facial erythema will be and the longer it will last. In addition, fair-skinned patients stay erythematous longer than darker-skinned patients, who have a greater propensity for transient dyspigmentation with the remote possibility of permanent hypopigmentation.

OTHER RESURFACING LASERS

The erbium:yttrium-aluminum-garnet (Er:YAG) laser has a 2,940-μm wavelength and produces energy in the midinfrared invisible light spectrum. This wavelength has 10 to 15 times the affinity for water absorption as the CO_2 laser (10,600 nm). This affinity for water produces tissue abla-

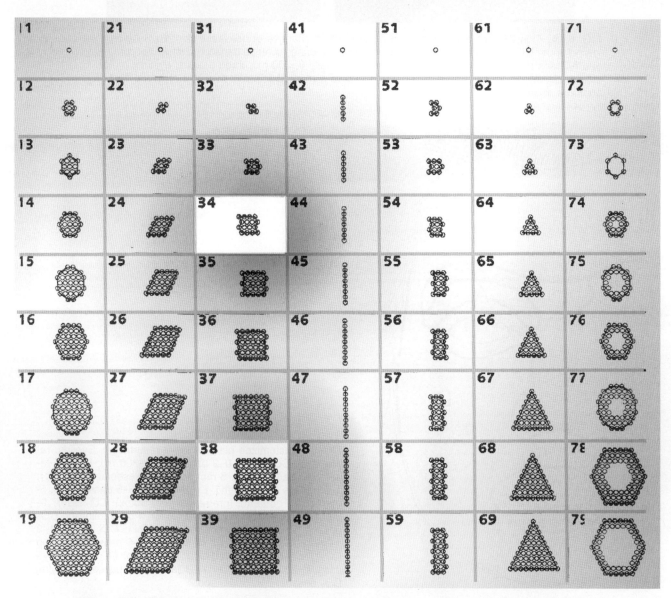

FIG. 8. Pattern 3, size 4, density 5 or 6 is used for resurfacing the eyelids, with power ranging from 150 to 300 mJ, depending on the desired degree of rhytid ablation or tissue tightening.

tion without vaporization and penetrates 15 to 25 μm per laser impact. This is much less penetration than the CO_2 laser (100 μm), causing less thermal damage. This translates into a shorter duration of postresurfacing erythema and a shorter recovery time. Posttreatment crusting has been described as lasting 2 to 7 days, with erythema lasting an average of 5.2 days. But it also means more passes of laser applications are necessary, and this treatment will not work on deep wrinkles or extensive photodamage. Spot sizes of 5 mm and 8 mm are used with powers of 1 to 2 J.

For segmental facial resurfacing, the Er:YAG laser can be applied without subcutaneous infiltration, utilizing topical tetracaine 4% gel (spread onto the skin 20 minutes before the procedure and left without an occlusive dressing) and supplemented with tetracaine 4% spray between passes. The slower the rate of laser application (passes per second),

the more easily tolerated it is by the patient (four to eight pulses per second).

Using a 5-mm spot and 1 J, at least four to five passes are needed to treat the crow's-feet area, and seven to eight passes are needed for most of the face. Fewer passes will be necessary if the power is increased to 2 J. Because there is no char, the skin does not have to be wiped between laser applications.

Clearly, this laser will fit into the total picture of facial rejuvenation. There are many patients with more superficial rhytids who can benefit from its use, without the inconvenience of intravenous sedation or local infiltration. In addition, it can be used as the final pass after CO_2 laser resurfacing to clearly ablate any residual debris without any additional thermal effect. Other creative combinations of lasers used for facial rejuvenation have yet to be described.

CHAPTER 13

Minimal-incision Facial Rejuvenation of the Lower Face and Neck ("Facelift Bypass"), Endoscopic Brow Lift, and Other Facial Endoscopic Procedures

Steven B. Hopping and Gregory Chernoff

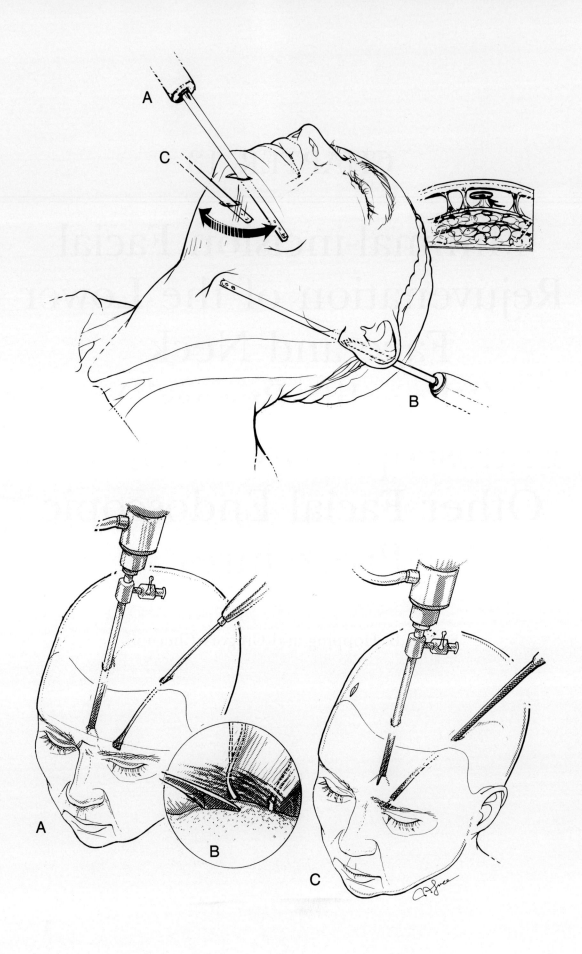

Many patients are interested in improving contour and aging changes of the lower two-thirds of the face, but they are not ready for facelift surgery, either psychologically or aesthetically. This might include younger persons with microgenia, early jowls, and submental fullness; men reluctant to sport preauricular surgical scars; or those who do not have the recovery time or resources required for an advanced facelift procedure. Minimal-incision techniques are available for this frequently encountered patient population. Among the most common of these procedures are neck and jowl liposuction with or without chin augmentation, buccal fat extraction, malar or submalar augmentation and microlipoaugmentation. These procedures can be accomplished through minimal-incision surgery and are characterized by absent or minimally visible scars, rapid recovery, and low risk.

SUBMENTAL AND JOWL LIPOSUCTION/LIPOSCULPTURE

Submental liposuction is indicated in patients whose major concern is fullness of the submental region or double chin. An additional concern of these patients may be early jowl formation. The ideal patient has a significant deposit of submental and neck fat with minimal platysmal banding and minimal jowling. If this patient also has microgenia, the combination of mentoplasty and neck liposuction can be quite dramatic (Fig. 1A,B). Many patients, however, benefit in varying degrees from neck and jowl liposuction alone. Young patients may complain of early neck and jowl laxity. Others may be looking for interim improvement prior to facelifting. The major advantage of the procedure is its minimal risk and minimal downtime. The major disadvantages are the limited tightening effect and the possibility of exposing platysma muscle banding. Nonetheless, the risk–benefit ratio is wide, and many patients are highly satisfied with properly performed neck and jowl liposculpting (Fig. 2A,B).

The procedure is easily performed utilizing local or light sedation anesthesia. A proper operating environment with pulse oximeter, blood pressure monitoring, and cardiac and airway emergency equipment is of course essential. Tumescent anesthesia is utilized, and the Kline formula with bicarbonate works well (Table 1). The concentration of epinephrine in the tumescent mixture can be increased to 2 mg/1 L of saline for facial liposuction and lipoharvesting to achieve greater hemostasis. The standard Kline tumescent formula, however, is quite adequate and well tolerated as a local procedure. It is important to wait at least 20 minutes to achieve maximum anesthetic and vasoconstrictive effect before surgery is begun. The tumescent anesthesia is injected with a 22-gauge needle or 1-mm blunt cannula utilizing a 10-mL syringe attached to an intravenous bag with a three-way stopcock.

One should start with a 1- or 2-mm rotator cannula (Fig. 3). Syringe technique or wall or machine suction are all effective. Generally, we perform this procedure with standard wall suction. Starting with a small cannula is especially important for the jowl region to prevent neuropraxia or damage to the ramus mandibularis branch of the facial nerve. Next, the operator should utilize a 2- or 3-mm cannula and follow the safe tunnels already created with the smaller rotator cannulas. It is important not to oversuction the fat on the flap side or skin side to prevent flap thinning, which can promote visualization of platysma bands. We prefer a spatula-type cannula, with the opening directed away from the skin while allowing maximal fat removal from the surface of the platysma muscle. The flat spatula cannula is also ideal for open liposuction technique. The liposuction procedure should initially be started through the submental incision and progress across and down the neck in a radial fashion, extending beyond the sternocleidomastoid muscle borders laterally and to the clavicles inferiorly. The surgeon must always be cognizant of the course of the ramus mandibularis nerve, when crossing the mandible. A 1-mm rotator cannula should be used to start, and one can

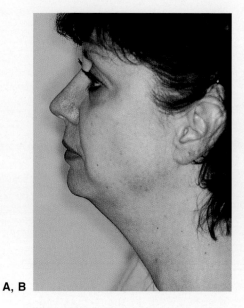
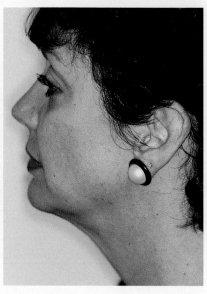

FIG. 1. A: Before. **B:** After chin augmentation (size-2 wrap-around anatomic Silastic chin implant) and neck and jowl liposuction. (Courtesy of Steven Hopping, M.D.)

A, B

then move to a 2-mm rotator cannula or the 3-mm spatula-type cannula.

Next, a 2-mm cannula is placed via a small midline stab incision into the subplatysmal plane. Often, fat can be identified in this subplatysmal area and its removal will further debulk the midline submentum, or double chin. Generally, only a few milliliters of fat are encountered, but the improved result is well worth the effect. Liposuction in the subplatysmal plane should be gentle and should be performed only in the midline to avoid injury to any neural or vascular structures.

TABLE 1. *Tumescent solution*

1 L normal saline 0.9
50 mL lidocaine 1% plain
1 mL epinephrine 1:1,000

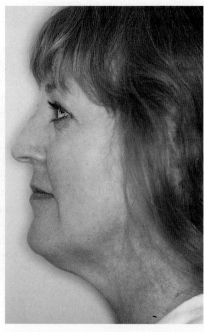
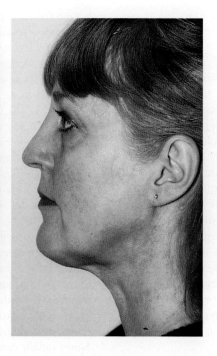

FIG. 2. A: Before: patient with neck and jowl fullness. **B:** After minimal-incision neck/jowl and subplatysmal liposuction, there is significant improvement. Note the skin tightening. (Courtesy of Steven Hopping, M.D.)

A, B

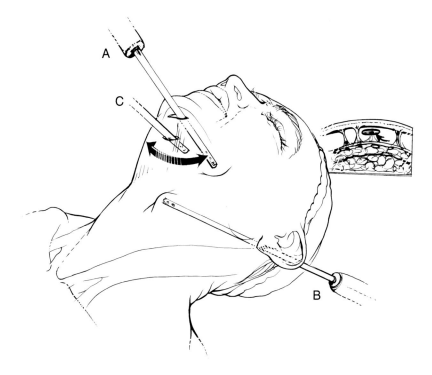

FIG. 3. Artist's depiction of the direction and plane of liposuction. Liposculpting of the neck and jowls was performed using 1- and 2-mm cannulas. **A:** Note the direction from the submental incision to access the neck and the jowl region. **B:** The cannula is passed through a sublobular incision to the neck, fanning out from the jowl down to the sternocleidomastoid muscle. **C:** A 2-mm cannula is placed into the subplatysmal space in the midline through a small stab incision in the platysma muscle. Often, additional fat can be accessed here, and its elimination will give patients a significantly improved result. The skin portal for cannula C would be the same as that for cannula A.

The lateral incisions are next placed just posterior and superior to the lower limits of each earlobe. A no. 11 blade is ideal for this incision. Again, a 1-mm rotator cannula is used to start the suctioning of the jowl and neck inferior to the mandibular border (see Fig. 3). Next, the 2-mm cannula is used, paralleling the mandibular border, again being careful not to oversuction. These maneuvers sculpt the mandibular border, sharpen the mandibular angle, and reduce fullness of the jowl. Finally, with the 2-mm cannula, the surgeon sweeps radially toward the sternocleidomastoid muscle, thereby crisscrossing the previous midline tunneling.

Visual inspection from the side and palpation of the neck with the pinch test assure symmetry and minimize irregularities. The tissues are moistened to permit enhanced tactile examination of the neck and jowls. Areas of palpable thickening or lumpiness are broken up or suctioned further.

The submental incision is then closed with a single nylon or 6-0 self-dissolving suture. The earlobe incisions are left open to promote drainage. A compressive dressing and/or grommet is placed. The patient is advised that the earlobe incisions might drain serosanguinous fluid for the first 6 to 12 hours.

The average amount of fat removed with neck and jowl liposuction is often only approximately 10 to 15 mL. The desired aesthetic result is one of debulking and tightening of the submental tissues. This is achieved not only by the fat removal but, more important, by the creation of multiple tunnels that heal as a fibrous web achieving internal tightening of the neck and jowl. This process evolves over the first 3 to 6 postoperative months. Patients are counseled to

massage the neck superiorly and posteriorly, which helps soften and smooth these fibrous tunnels as they heal. The resultant subcutaneous fibrous network is long lasting and can effectively improve mild to moderate neck laxity. Removed fat cells will never return, and in this sense the procedure has permanence.

CHIN AUGMENTATION

Chin augmentation can greatly enhance the results of neck liposuction and should always be considered and encouraged if indicated. Patients with microgenia should always be offered the option of mentoplasty when neck and jowl liposuction is planned. The result of these combined procedures is often dramatic (Fig. 4A,B). Strengthening of the chin with chin augmentation extends the cervical neckline and allows better draping of the neck skin following liposuction, or rhytidectomy for that matter. Chin augmentation can be performed through the same submental incision as that used for liposuction. Our implant material of choice is extended, solid Silastic (preformed anatomic implants).

Following neck and jowl liposuction, the submental incision is extended slightly, approximately 1 to 1.5 cm. Sharp dissection is directed superiorly toward the mentum. A supraperiosteal pocket is created over the midline mentum, with care taken to preserve the periosteal integrity at the inferior mandibular border. We feel this limits bone resorption and provides soft tissue available for securing the implant in the desired position to the inferior mandibular margin. Laterally, along the inferior borders of the mandible, subperiosteal

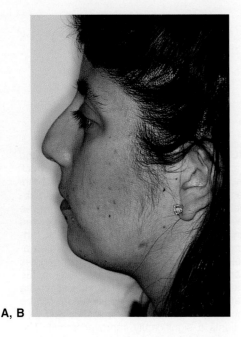
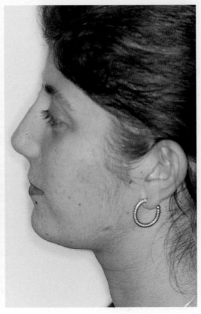

FIG. 4. A: Before. **B:** After chin augmentation (size 2 anatomic Silastic chin implant) and neck liposuction. (Courtesy of Steven Hopping, M.D.)

A, B

pockets are created to allow placement of the lateral wings or extensions of the anatomically styled implants. By hugging the inferior border of the mandible, one can be certain to avoid injury to the mental nerves as they exit from the mental foramen more superiorly, at the level of the first premolar tooth. Maintaining a subperiosteal plane also prevents injury to the ramus mandibularis nerve (Fig. 5).

Various sizers can be used to assist in the selection of the proper implant (Fig. 6). Once selected, the implant is inserted into the right subperiosteal tunnel with a curved

hemostat. Next, the left subperiosteal tunnel is located with a Senn retractor, and the free end of the implant is fed into the tunnel, again with the assistance of a hemostat. The implant should move freely, right and left, and be free of tension as it sits in the created pocket.

If there is tension or if the implant does not move freely, either the pocket must be enlarged or the implant downsized. Implants should rest evenly along the inferior border of the mandible without bowing. A 4-0 Vicryl suture secures the implant to the mandibular periosteum, assuring

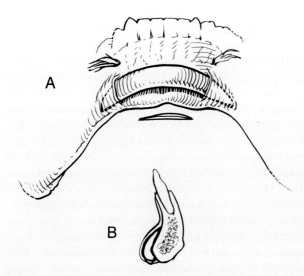

FIG. 5. A: The chin implant must be properly placed along the inferior border of the mandible. The lateral portion of the implants is placed subperiosteally. The implant lying over the mentum is supraperiosteal. The incision is submental. **B:** Lateral view shows the proper placement of the implant in relation to the alveolar bone and dentition.

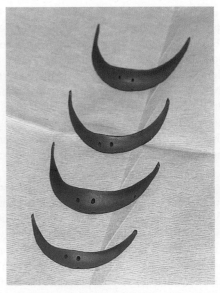

FIG. 6. Anatomic chin implant sizers: sizes 1 through 4. (Courtesy of Steven Hopping, M.D.)

its position at the inferior border. One or two sutures are utilized. The wound is then copiously irrigated with saline or saline/antibiotic solution, and then three 4-0 Vicryl sutures are used to close the muscular defect. This layer of closure seals the implant and controls most of the bleeding encountered with this operation. The skin can then be closed with either 5-0 nylon or a 6-0 self-absorbing suture. Improvement is immediately apparent on the table. Rarely is an intraoral approach selected, since generally some amount of neck liposuction is usually performed with chin augmentation. The intraoral approach is also associated with a significantly higher infection rate and a tendency for the implant to rise into the genioalveolar sulcus, which is unwanted.

Complications of chin augmentation include transient hypesthesia and transient muscle weakness that can affect smile symmetry. Fortunately, these two complications are generally self-limiting and improve with time. Persistent hypesthesia must be addressed, and the implant should be checked to ensure that there is no pressure on the mental nerve. Infection is always a concern and is certainly significantly less frequent with the submental approach than the intraoral approach. Any implant that becomes infected is best removed, and the wound cultured and treated appropriately; then consideration can be given for implant replacement in 6 to 8 weeks. Signs of implant infection are intermittent swelling, tenderness, and occasionally erythema. This may occur within the first 10 days of surgery, but it may also be seen in a delayed fashion some weeks or months following the procedure. Staphylococci are most often responsible, and prophylactic antibiotic therapy should be appropriately directed.

MALAR/SUBMALAR MIDFACE AUGMENTATION

Malar or submalar augmentation can often correct midfacial aging or atrophy without resorting to midface lifting or anterior rhytidectomy. Fullness in the malar and submalar areas is a youthful trait that diminishes with age, principally due to soft tissue atrophy and medial-inferior soft tissue displacement. Restoring fullness to the atrophic midface with malar/submalar augmentation is one of the most dramatic and most long lasting of all cosmetic procedures. Individuals blessed with high cheekbones generally age more favorably than their counterparts. Malar or midface enhancement is also indicated in patients with congenital malar hypoplasia. Many of these patients complain of a sad look, and indeed correction with midface augmentation can reverse this undesirable feature. The alloplast of choice for midfacial augmentation is solid Silastic rubber. This firm implant mimics the cheekbone density and readily adheres to the malar bone. Our current implants of choice are the Binder submalar implant (XoMed, Boston, MA) and the Terino malar shell (XoMed, Boston, MA) (Fig. 7). These implants are nicely feathered, particularly the Terino, and can be easily camouflaged by the overlying cheek soft tissue. The submalar implant is selected in a patient requiring more medial augmentation. The shell is suitable for patients desiring more diffuse cheek fullness or more lateral, higher profile enhancement. Both implants, as mentioned, are feathered laterally, but the Terino shell is a better choice for extremely thin-faced or gaunt patients (Fig. 8A,B).

The approach of choice is the buccal or oral approach, utilizing bilateral 2-cm horizontal incisions just lateral to the maxillary canine teeth. The incisions are placed high in the sulcus, but a ledge of gingival mucosa must be preserved for closure. Adjustments in the level of the incision should be made in denture wearers to avoid irritation from the appliance. Therefore, the denture is left in place so that the proper level of incision can be ascertained.

All patients are instructed preoperatively to rinse with chlorhexidine gluconate (Peridex) 3 days prior to surgery. All patients receive cefazolin sodium, 1 g intramuscularly or intravenously, just prior to surgery and are maintained on cephalexin, 500 mg three times a day, for 5 days following the surgery. The incisional area is prepared with povidone-iodine prior to the procedure.

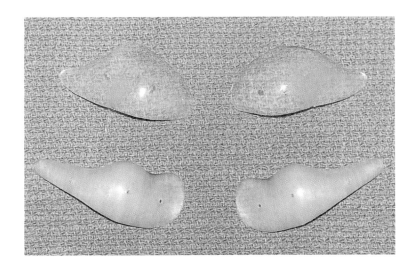

FIG. 7. In cheek augmentation, the Terino shell and Binder midfacial implant are both feathered for optimal contouring. (Courtesy of Steven Hopping, M.D.)

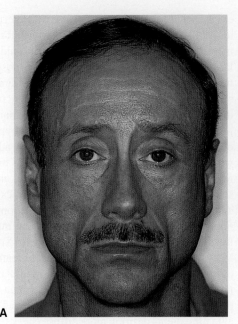 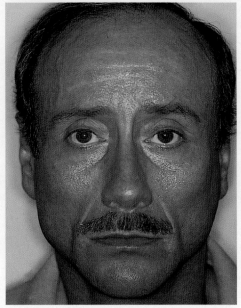

A   B

FIG. 8. A: Before: thin-faced man with little soft tissue in the malar area. **B:** After augmentation, large Terino shell implants fill the malar depressions. These implants are feathered to mask their appearance in thin patients. (Courtesy of Steven Hopping, M.D.)

Following a deliberate incision down to the bone, the level of dissection is immediately in the subperiosteal plane. This safe, bloodless plane is continued over the front face of the malar bone toward the zygomatic arch. A Joseph or Key elevator works well for this dissection. At the level of the zygomatic arch, however, sharp dissection is required to sever strong periosteal attachments and lift the soft tissue envelope. Medially, the infraorbital nerve is identified and avoided. Blunt dissection with Metzenbaum scissors with the blades slightly apart is often helpful in freeing any remaining soft tissue attachments. A moist gauze is then packed into the pocket, which can give the surgeon a sense of the pocket size and extent. With the gauze in place, the opposite side is similarly developed. Comparing the dimensions of the packed gauze bilaterally gives the surgeon an idea of pocket symmetry.

Various implants or sizers are fitted to allow selection of the one that provides the desired contours. After the most appropriate implant is selected, a 5-0 nylon suture is threaded through the high point or widest dimension of the implant. The desired high point of the implant has already been marked with a marking pen on the skin of the patient when the patient is smiling in a sitting position. This point should be exactly the same bilaterally. For patients desiring a more lateral enhancement, the point is marked accordingly. Using curved or angled Keith needles, the two ends of the nylon suture that had been brought through the implant are then passed through the elevated periosteum, soft tissue, and skin at exactly the desired high point level. The suture is then tied firmly over a bolster dressing. We often use a quarter-size piece of medium thick, medium soft Si-

lastic sheeting to protect the skin, but a dental roll works just as efficiently (Fig. 9).

The incision is then copiously irrigated with saline or an antibiotic solution and closed with 4-0 chromic sutures. The knots can be buried to give added patient comfort. A two-layer closure, although desirable, is often difficult and, in our experience, not essential.

The bolster dressing provides stability and fixes the position of the implants quite exactly. The bolster dressing also reduces the likelihood of hematoma and seroma formation. The bolster suture and dressing are removed on the third postoperative day. The implant should be stable and fixed at that point. If there is palpable fluid, this should be drained sterilely under local anesthesia with an 18-gauge angiocatheter via the gingival buccal sulcus. Antibiotic therapy can be extended if either or both of the implants are floating or if one suspects seroma or incipient infection.

The fixation or bolster dressing helps minimize the major complications with cheek augmentation: asymmetry, seroma or hematoma formation, implant movement, and infection. Other potential complications are hyperesthesia or anesthesia, palpable implant edges, pain, and implant extrusion, particularly if an infection occurs. The best policy regarding frank infection is to remove the involved implant or implants, culture the wound, treat with the appropriate antibiotic, and consider replacing the implant(s) in 6 to 8 weeks. Once a clinical infection has occurred around an implant, it is rare that antibiotics can resolve the situation without implant removal. In our experience, cheek implant infections occur in less than 5% of procedures.

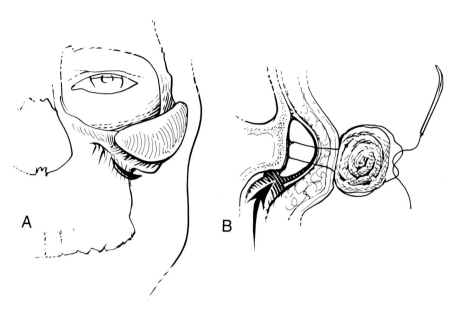

FIG. 9. A: The malar cheek implant is correctly placed when it follows the contour of the normal malar bone. **B:** Artist's depiction shows proper fixation of the malar implant using transcutaneous sutures tied over a bolster dressing. This secures the implant, thereby minimizing asymmetry and hematoma and seroma formation.

AUTOLOGOUS MICROLIPOAUGMENTATION (FAT TRANSFERS)

Microaugmentation is a very low-risk, high-yield technique for improving early signs of atrophic aging (Figs. 10A,B, 11A,B). This includes filling glabellar frown lines, midfacial smile lines, and lower facial marionette grooves (Fig. 12A,B). Fat transfers can enhance the other minimal-incision facelift bypass procedures already described. Fat is best harvested from the lower extremities—lateral thigh, knee, or buttocks. Fat harvested from the abdomen can often be somewhat bloody, but nonetheless this area can be a donor area in selected patients. Fat harvested from the neck is usually scant and somewhat fibrous in nature.

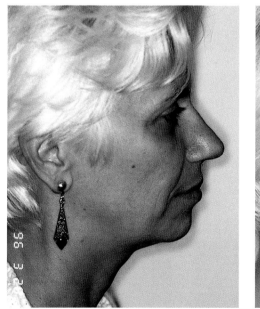
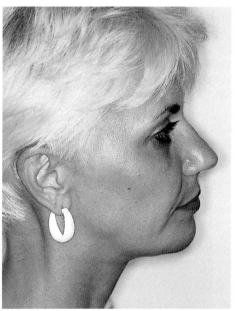

FIG. 10. A: Before. **B:** After cheek augmentation with medium Binder implants, chin augmentation with a medium anatomic implant, neck liposuction, and fat transfers to smile, frown, and marionette lines. (Courtesy of Steven Hopping, M.D.)

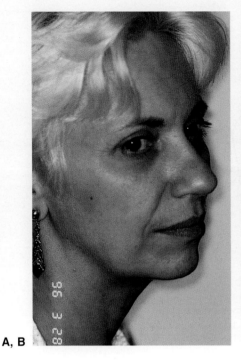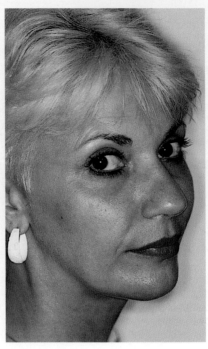

FIG. 11. A: Before. **B:** After "facelift bypass:" cheek and chin augmentation, neck and jowl liposuction, and fat transfers. (Courtesy of Steven Hopping, M.D.)

The donor area is injected with the same tumescent solution used for neck liposuction (see Table 1). It is important to allow a 10- to 20-minute interval to achieve maximum hemostasis and anesthesia prior to harvesting the fat. Harvesting is most easily accomplished with a 14-gauge blunt cannula with one or two small ports. The cannula is attached to 10-mL syringes, which provide the best system for collecting fat. An attempt is made to harvest between 40 and 50 mL of fat at each harvesting session. We always plan a series of at least three fat transfer sessions spaced approximately 4 to 6 weeks apart to achieve maximum improvement.

The 10-mL syringes are placed into a test tube pipe stand oriented vertically to allow the fat and supernatant blood and fluid to separate. The fat is washed with the same tumescent solution until all visible red blood cells are gone. This is easily accomplished by adding 2 mL of the same tumescent solution

to the fat and then turning the syringe back and forth to rinse the fat with the saline. It is again placed in the vertical position to allow separation. After the fat is clean and has floated to the top and separated from the fluid and red blood cells, the supernatant is discarded from the syringe, leaving only cleansed fat. The fat is then transferred to 3-mL syringes, with a syringe transfer adapter allowing a no-touch technique. The 3-mL syringes allow controlled fat injection through an 18-gauge needle or blunt cannula. Utilizing the 18-gauge blunt cannula/3-mL syringe system permits the safe placement of small aliquots of fat at literally any level anywhere on the face. Fat can be layered just above the periosteum, into the muscle, and subcutaneously without fear of lacerating a vessel or damaging a nerve. One can safely treat tear-trough depressions without concern for the infraorbital nerve, or inject into the glabellar frown lines without consideration of lacerating

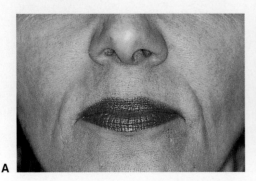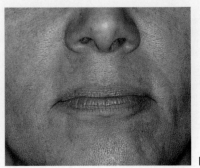

FIG. 12. A: Before: young woman with premature deep myolabial folds. **B:** After two sessions of autologous fat transfers (3 mL to each side each session), there is improvement. (Courtesy of Steven Hopping, M.D.)

a supratrochlear vessel. It is important to inject small quantities of fat, 0.25 to 0.5 mL, in multiple areas. Conceptually, successful microlipotransfers create multiple, isolated puddles of fat, not lakes.

Keeping this concept in mind will help maximize the number of fat cells achieving vascularity and therefore viability. On the average, 5 mL of fat is placed in each cheek, 2 mL in the glabellar frown lines, 3 mL in the smile lines, 1 to 2 mL in the marionette lines, and 2 to 4 mL in each of the upper and lower lips. An 18-gauge NoKor needle is ideal for creating an entrance site for the 18-gauge cannula. It is not necessary to suture the incision left with the NoKor needle, and it heals quite inconspicuously, as compared to a no. 11 or no. 15 blade incision. The remaining fat is double-sealed in plastic bags, labeled, dated, and placed alphabetically in a freezer solely designated for fat storage. We use a small 3- × 3-foot freezer and store the fat of 50 to 60 patients at any one time. A series of three lipotransfers or fat injection sessions is scheduled, usually 4 to 6 weeks apart. If we anticipate at least a 30% survival with each treatment, three such treatments should translate into approximately a 90% correction rate. Obviously, some patients seem to have better long-term fat survivability than others. There is no question, however, that long-term correction of vertical smile, frown and marionette

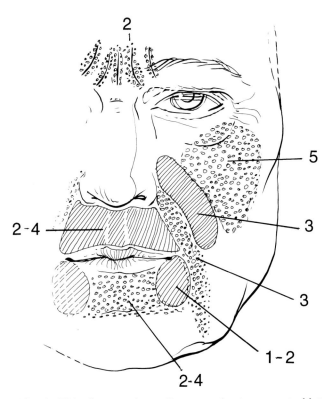

FIG. 13. This diagram shows the approximate amount of fat in fat-transfer procedures: 5 mL to the cheek, 2 to 3 mL in the smile line, 1 to 2 mL in the marionette groove, 2 to 4 mL in the upper and lower lips, and 1 to 2 mL in the glabella. Again, it is important to place small aliquots of fat rather than to create a large "fat lake."

lines, tear-trough depressions, and hypoplastic cheeks and lips can be achieved (Fig. 13).

BUCCAL FAT PAD EXTRACTION

Partial extraction of the body of the buccal fat pad is another effective minimal-incision procedure for patients with excessively round or jowly lower faces. Removing a portion of the body of the buccal fat pad, or the fat pad of Bichet, can debulk the jowl and the lower cheek in these cherubic individuals. Patients with strong cheekbones and round faces are particularly good candidates for buccal fat extraction (Figs. 14A,B, 15A,B) The procedure should be avoided in young patients who may lose their baby fat as they mature into adulthood.

The procedure is usually performed under local anesthesia. A 50/50 mixture of lidocaine 1% with 1:100,000 epinephrine solution mixed equally with bupivacaine 0.25% with 1:200,000 epinephrine solution and buffered with bicarbonate works well. The local is infiltrated into the gingival buccal sulci with a 1.5-inch, 27-gauge needle. The injection fluid is diffused toward the buccal space. Approximately 5 to 6 mL of local anesthesia is used on each side. The patient should be supine, parallel to the floor, with the head slightly elevated. A 1.5-cm incision is made in the mucosa of the gingival buccal sulcus at the level of the first premolar tooth. Blunt dissection is then directed inferiorly between the mucosa and the hard maxillary bone, with gentle spreading of the Metzenbaum scissors creating a plane of dissection to the buccal space. The tips of the scissors can be felt penetrating the thin membrane leading into the buccal space. Gentle upward and medial pressure on the jowl by an assistant will encourage the buccal fat pad to emerge into the wound. Retraction is best accomplished with an Aufrecht retractor. The buccal fat pad should always be approached from the medial surface. The buccal branches of the facial nerve run on the lateral surface of the fat pad, and approaching the fat medially avoids inadvertent injury to these facial nerve branches. The buccal fat is whitish-yellow and has a thin capsule, not unlike the medial orbital fat pad (Fig. 16).

After identification of the fat pad, it should be teased out of the buccal space with DeBakey forceps. The assistant should also grasp the fat pad as the surgeon progressively and gently removes a portion of the body of the fat pad of Bichet. Any vessels encountered should be cauterized with a bipolar cautery. Equal amounts of buccal fat from both sides should be removed. After removal of the fat pad, the decrease in bulkiness of the jowl and lower cheek is immediately noticed and can be appreciated both visually and with palpation. The endpoint of fat pad removal should be determined by the amount of debulking achieved and symmetrical reductions. The incision is then closed with a single 4-0 chromic suture. The blunt curved scissor, the Aufrecht retractor, and the DeBakey forceps are utilized for buccal fat extraction.

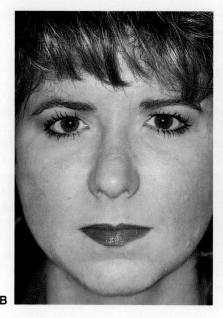
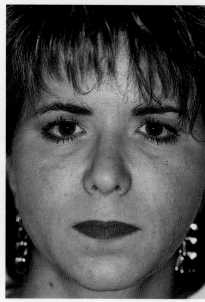

A, B

FIG. 14. A: Before buccal fat extraction. **B:** After buccal fat extraction. (Courtesy of Steven Hopping, M.D.)

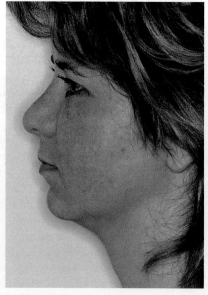
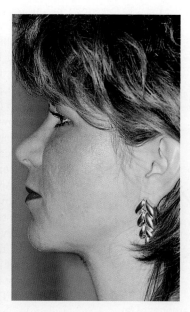

A, B

FIG. 15. A: Before. **B:** After buccal fat extraction, chin augmentation, and neck liposuction, note illusion of higher cheekbones. (Courtesy of Steven Hopping, M.D.)

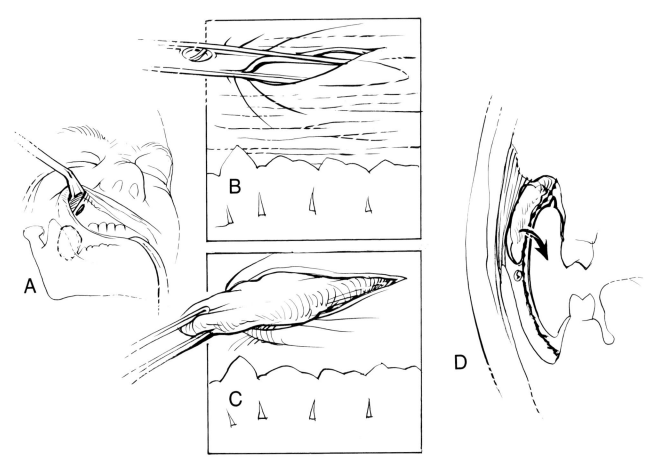

FIG. 16. The excision of buccal fat pad: **(A)** horizontal gingival buccal incision, **(B)** blunt dissection to buccal fat, **(C)** gentle teasing to remove buccal fat, **(D)** approaching the fat pad medially to avoid facial injury.

Possible complications include hematoma, infection, asymmetry, and weakness of the upper lip secondary to injury to the buccal branches of the facial nerve. Again, facial nerve injury is avoided by always approaching and handling the buccal fat pad from the medial surface.

ENDOSCOPIC AESTHETIC PLASTIC SURGICAL APPROACHES

The field of aesthetic plastic surgery continues to be one of the most creative and innovative of the surgical specialties. This is fed by patients' desire to undergo minimally invasive procedures with minimal risk, minimal pain, and minimal healing time while yielding maximal benefit. The advent of microchip technology and improved optics allows surgeons to make diagnoses and surgically address situations that previously required larger incisions. Increased precision and accuracy through smaller incisions theoretically yields less pain and shorter recovery times. Minimal-incision techniques require an in-depth knowledge of the microanatomy of the situation at hand. As these techniques continue to evolve, surgical creativity must not mask patient safety. Objective studies must be performed to critically evaluate surgical outcomes to ensure that the minimally invasive approaches yield equal quality to previously time-tested procedures.

Endoscopic procedures have opened collaborative efforts among multiple specialties, as well as equipment providers such as laser companies, imaging companies, and endoscopic equipment companies. These collaborative efforts have spurred fascinating studies and will continue to further advance this ever growing field.

Patient selection is by far the most important criterion for success of these procedures. Appropriate evaluation of the aging face begins with dividing the face into thirds. The upper one-third of the face consists of the region between the hairline and the glabella, the middle one-third extends from the glabella to the subnasal region, and the lower one-third comprises the subnasal region to the menton of the chin. The neck is usually involved with evaluation of the lower one-third of the face. As gravitational forces take hold, the brows fall, blepharochalasis and dermatochalasis appear, and the midface falls, with subsequent deepening of the nasolabial and melolabial folds.

Gravity then plays havoc with the lower one-third of the face, yielding jowling and submental fullness. Quantitative or gravitational signs of aging should not be confused with qualitative signs of aging of the skin. With aging, skin loses its moisture and elasticity. Redistribution of fat is coupled with muscle atrophy. Resorption of the bony skeleton also occurs.

It is now possible to approach each third of the face with endoscopic approaches.

Endoscopic Forehead and Brow Lift

No other third of the face is as dynamic and expressive as the upper one-third. This region serves as a focus for expression of emotion and personality and is often the first area to exhibit the changes of aging. The basic concept of the endoscopic forehead and brow lift involves a dynamic, functional repositioning of the eye brow and forehead. Brow ptosis results from weakening of the frontalis muscle, while increased glabellar rhytids result from weakened depressor muscles, including the corrugator supercilii, the procerus, and the depressor supercilii muscles and the orbital portion of the orbicularis oculi muscles.

Before the decision is made as to whether excess blepharo- or dermatochalasis will be dealt with, effective management of the ptotic brow is crucial. Ptosis of the brow can contribute to superior and lateral visual-field defects. Excess weight in this region may also interfere with upper eyelid motility. The head-to-tail relationship of the eyebrow is a relationship that gauges physical appearance, as well as projection of one's mood. The benefit of an endoscopic approach to the eyebrows is that the head-to-tail relationship can be modified to within millimeters to achieve the desired results. For example, brows that have close heads yield a masculine scowling appearance, while a downwardly wrapped tail of the brow reveals a saddened appearance (Fig. 17A,B).

Cephalometric parameters are helpful in considering each patient. McKinney suggested that the normal distance from the midpupil to the upper brow is 2.5 cm. A lesser distance is a possible indication for foreheadplasty or brow lift. Farcus noted that the acceptable distance from the trichion to the glabellar area should be approximately 6 cm, and from the brow to the anterior hairline, 5 cm. If measurements are less than those aforementioned, foreheadplasty is also indicated.

Sasaki proposed two useful parameters for making the selection of the appropriate surgical maneuver for each particular patient. The frame height is the distance between the midpupil and the top of the brow, with the patient sitting in a relaxed position and with the eyes looking straight ahead. The procedure for making this determination is identical to that performed by McKinney. The distance from the midpupil to the top of the central brow ranges from 2 to 2.5 cm. The glide test measures the degree of brow ptosis by recording the maximal upward excursion of the medial, central, and lateral portions of the eyebrow from a neutral resting position, with the patient sitting in the upright position. If the glide test results are less than 1.2 cm, then the surgical maneuver selected includes wide undermining, orbicularis oculi muscle myotomies laterally, and frontal and temporal fixation, plus treatment of muscle hyperactivity. If the glide test results are greater than 1.2 cm, then the surgical maneuver should include wide undermining and frontal and temporal fixation, plus treatment of muscle hyperactivity only if it is present.

The endoscopic method of forehead and brow surgery entails combining three basic methods to alter the forehead. The first technique involves myotomy of the small facial muscles that depress the brow, including the corrugator, procerus, depressor, and orbicularis, with elevation of the frontalis muscle. Second, shifting the forehead backward in relation to the rest of the skull also elevates the eyebrows. These procedures act to elevate the eyebrows, reduce hor-

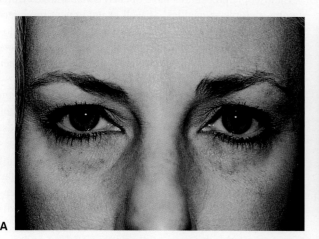 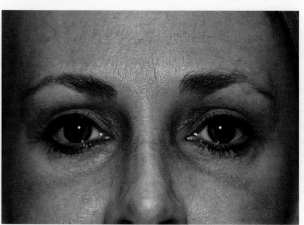

FIG. 17. A: Before: brow ptosis with secondary redundant upper lid folds. **B:** After endoscopic brow lift, upper lid blepharoplasty and transconjunctival lower lid blepharoplasty. (Courtesy of Gregory Chernoff, M.D.)

izontal forehead rhytids and vertical glabellar rhytids, elevate any lateral canthal hooding, and also reduce the infrabrow skin overhang produced by the gravitational forces of the forehead tissues in the region of the brow body.

The minimally invasive nature of the endoscopic technique involves the following:

- Small, inconspicuous incisions
- Tissue undermining of the forehead, scalp, and temporal areas
- Tissue mobilization and modification
- Tissue advancement and redraping
- Fixation methods

Theory behind Consistency

Through the use of small, multiple incisions, access is gained to the forehead for both the endoscope and the other instruments used. Coronal and pretrichial approaches have been notorious for damage to the supraorbital sensory nerves. Accompanying alopecia was also a problem. Variations of the small-incision approach are tailored for hair-loss patterns, surgical access, and forehead size.

Basic incision placement can be divided proportionally to whether the patient requires less than 1-cm elevation or greater than 1-cm elevation of the tail of the brow. If less than 1-cm elevation is required, three incisions can be utilized to perform the procedure. These three incisions encompass one horizontal central incision and two vertical incisions placed at the level of the lateral limbus over the frontal bone. The lateral incision placement keeps the incisions closest to the region of the tail of the brow to gain maximal upward pull at this region. If the patient requires greater than 1-cm elevation, six incisions are utilized. The first three incisions are as previously mentioned, with the addition of diagonally placed temporal incisions with the bottom portion of the incision at the superior orbital rim. This placement permits maximal outward and upward force on the brow tail. The sixth incision is then placed at the superior portion of the occipital bone to facilitate posterior dissection to the level of the posterior occipital arteries.

Male-pattern Baldness

Patients with male-pattern baldness require variation of the incisions. For men, 1-cm vertical incisions placed along the male fringe are acceptable. With a small vertical incision, the frontal tuft can be utilized: If a frontal tuft will be created with hair transplantation techniques, a single 1-cm incision can also be placed in the midline. With absence of a frontal tuft, the frontal area can be accessed through a blepharoplasty incision in a retrograde fashion.

Women with high foreheads wishing to lower the hairline require a trichophytic incision or a pretrichial incision. Receding hairlines in women require utilization of a single vertical central incision, rather than two midcentral incisions, to access the midforehead region.

Temple incisions are perhaps the most important and can be varied proportionally to the tailoring required for specific patients. The outward vector of this incision allows not only elevating lateral hooding but also bringing the glabellar region upward and outward. The lateral limbal incision can also be varied more centrally to allow a more powerful medial brow pull.

Tissue Undermining

Since there is no natural cavity in the forehead in which to place an endoscope, the surgeon must create optical cavities for access of the instrumentation. Naturally occurring tissue planes existing in the forehead and temple can be utilized to facilitate these optical cavities. Options for the creation of optical cavities include the following planes:

- Subperiosteal
- Subgaleal
- Subcutaneous
- Composite of these three planes

The safest combination of the aforementioned planes includes anterior dissection in the subperiosteal plane with posterior dissection in the subgaleal plane. Dissection in the temporal region must be immediately on top of the deepest layer or temporal fascia to avoid injury to the temporal branch of the facial nerve, which sits in the fat pad lying between the middle and deep layers of the temporal fascia. The advantage of utilizing the subperiosteal plane is that it tends to be less vascular than the subcutaneous or subgaleal planes. The subperiosteal plane also allows a greater component of tissue for fixation purposes. A disadvantage of using the subperiosteal plane is that it is stiffer than the subgaleal and subcutaneous planes and therefore allows less stretch-back of the forehead, producing somewhat less elevation than dissection in the other two planes.

To access the musculature of the forehead, transition must be made into the subgaleal plane. This plane must also be entered if undermining is to be continued over the malar eminence for a midface lift. The subgaleal plane is preferred if less brow and forehead elevation is required. If greater brow elevation is required, the subperiosteal plane is preferred to minimize forehead elevation. In patients with short foreheads needing greater forehead lengthening, the subgaleal plane is also advantageous, especially if prominent horizontal rhytids are present.

The subcutaneous plane is less frequently utilized, but comes into play when the surgeon wishes to lower the forehead. Once again, transition can be made into the subgaleal plane for muscle modification. Pretrichial skin can be excised following advancement of the underlying frontalis muscle when the forehead is pulled backward.

Most commonly, an anterior subperiosteal dissection is created over the frontal bone to the level of the eyebrow. In the midline, at the level of the eyebrow, transition is made to a supraperiosteal plane over the nose between the insertions of the corrugator muscle. Access is then gained to the corrugator, procerus, depressor, and the orbicularis musculature in the subgaleal plane. This transition to the supraperiosteal plane is also made over the orbital rim on the descending zygomatic process onto the malar eminence. In the temple, the cavity is created over the superficial layer of deep temporal fascia. Joining of these two cavities is under direct vision in the endoscopic field. The primary reason for performing posterior dissection is to permit re-draping of the skin following backward fixation.

Tissue Mobilization and Modification

To facilitate elevation of the brow, the periosteum, muscles, and fascial connections acting to depress or bind the brow down to bone in proximity of the orbital rim must be released. This can be divided into three main regions: (a) medial to the supraorbital nerve bundles, (b) lateral to the supraorbital nerve bundles to the lateral orbital rim, and (c) lateral frontal release at the insertion of the temporal line and malar eminence.

The sequential release of the brow is facilitated through the use of laser fibers by greatly increasing hemostasis potential. The medial release involves the corrugator, procerus, orbicularis, and depressor muscles, innervated by a branch of the temporal facial nerve, as well as branches of the zygomatic nerve and buccal branches of the facial nerve. Incising these muscles near their bony attachment is essential to releasing the medial aspect of the brow. Some surgeons feel that incising the frontal branch of the facial nerve along the brow medial to the supraorbital nerve and lateral to the supratrochlear nerve is sufficient to elevate the medial brow.

Lateral to the supraorbital nerve, the periosteum is released below the bony orbital rim and then incised horizontally after entry into the retroorbicularis fat pad.

The lateral temporal portion of the brow is released by incising the conjoint tendon at the level of the brow, thus connecting the frontal and temporal cavities. To properly elevate the tail of the brow, release of tissues over the malar eminence is required.

Tissue Advancement and Redraping

Once all of the depressor muscles are released and the retaining periosteum and fibrous structures are freed, the surgeon is able to shift the scalp and underlying periosteum posteriorly. With this maneuver, the brows are elevated without excision of scalp. Redundancy of scalp soft tissue posterior to the fixation points is usually created on posterior shifting of the scalp. These small dog-ears usually disappear within weeks.

Tissue Fixation

Fixation is usually performed at the lateral canthal or lateral limbal incision, with possible fixation also per-formed at the central incision. The fixation of the scalp's new position to a point on the skull is accomplished through the use of screws, sutures, plates, or skin and scalp excision.

Basic Technique

The evolution of endoscopic brow-lifting procedures has shown tremendous refinements. Following a step-by-step, systematic approach with each patient allowing for anatomic variation is a key to consistency. Knowledge of the anatomy of the region to the millimeter is essential for both procedural success and avoidance of unacceptable complications during the procedure. The following approach permits such consistency.

Patient Preparation and Incisions

The endoscopic brow procedure is commonly performed under either MAC (monitored anesthetic control) or general anesthesia. The supraorbital notch and/or supratrochlear nerve are first palpated and marked (Fig. 18). The region encompassing 2 cm above the brow bilaterally delineates the position where blind undermining is not performed. Well over 10% of patients will have a supraorbital foramen, as opposed to a supraorbital notch.

The incisions are then marked (Fig. 19). The central incision should be made horizontally and, with increasing experience, can be converted to a vertical incision. The two lateral limbal incisions are fashioned, followed by the two temporal incisions and then by the superior occipital incision. Once again, if less than 1-cm elevation is required, the latter three incisions are not the purpose of this chapter. The central incision is made 2 cm long, with each remaining incision being 1.5 cm in length.

Before the incisions are made, lidocaine 1% with 1:100,000 epinephrine is infiltrated in the region of the incisions and the supraorbital bundles and along the course of the eyebrows bilaterally. Tumescent solution (see Table 1), is then injected over the entire surface to be undermined and dissected.

The central incision is made first, followed by the two incisions at the level of the lateral limbus. The incisions are taken down to the level of the periosteum, and the periosteum is secured to the incision's subcutaneous tissue to prevent periosteal injury with subsequent insertion and removal of equipment (Fig. 20). After the incisions at the lateral limbus level are made, a carbon dioxide laser is used to score the bone at the anterior-most portion of this incision. This scoring is used as a mark for the beginning of the procedure and will serve as a reference point for placement of the fixation plate. This lateral vector of pull is required at the lateral portion of the eyebrow. Next, the diagonal temple incisions are made, 2 cm in length and approximately 2 cm behind the hairline. The midpoint of these incisions is usually placed at a horizontal line con-

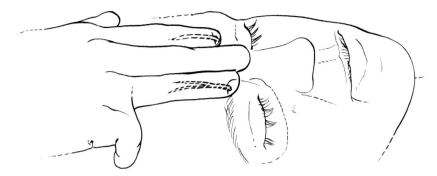

FIG. 18. Three-finger rule: denotes safe location of supraorbital bundle, with injection lateral to index and ring fingers. (Courtesy of Gregory Chernoff, M.D.)

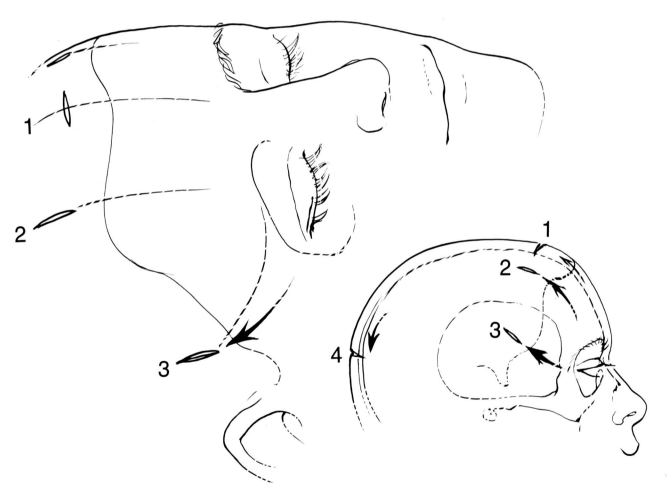

FIG. 19. Horizontal midline incision (*1*); vertical incision, lateral limbus level (*2*); and temporal incision 45 degrees to lateral canthus (*3*). (Courtesy of Gregory Chernoff, M.D.)

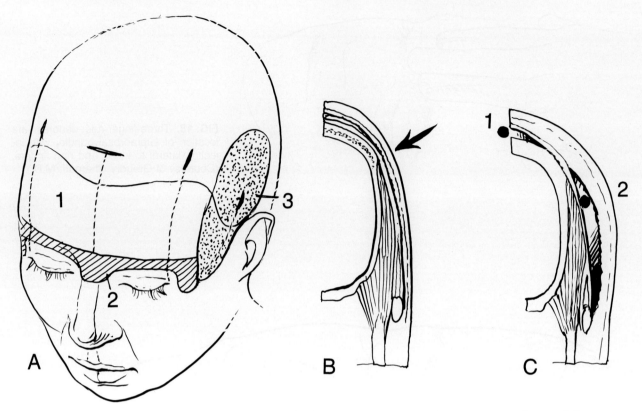

FIG. 20. Dissection planes: subperiosteal (*1*); division of corrugator and procerus muscles medially and arcus semilunaris bilaterally laterally (*2*); superficial to deep layer of temporalis fascia (*3*). (Courtesy of Gregory Chernoff, M.D.)

necting the two superior orbital rims. The superior occipital incision is made last.

Tissue Elevation

The instrumentation used in this procedure can be found in Table 2. Blind dissection is initially performed through the central and lateral canthal incisions to a level 2 cm above the supraorbital rims. The endoscope is then inserted through the central incision, and throughout the course of the procedure, it should not be removed from this incision (Fig. 21A–C).

The lateral limbal and lateral temporal incisions will then serve as the ports of entry for the endoscopic equipment.

(text continues on page 159)

TABLE 2. *Instrumentation used in endoscopic forehead and brow lift*

Storz catalogue number	Description
	PES instrument
N9000	Elevator
N9001	Dissector
N9002	Nerve hook, right
N9003	Nerve hook, left
N9004	Cannula, 4 mm
N9005	Separator, 18F
N9006	Separator, 20F
N9100	Grasping forceps, curved right
N9101	Grasping forceps, curved left
N9102	Punch, curved right
N9103	Punch, curved left
N9104	Scissors, straight
N9105	Scissors, curved down
N9106	Scissors, curved right

Continued next page

TABLE 2. *Continued.*

Storz catalogue number	Description
N9107	Scissors, curved left
	PES instrument set total
	PES endoscope system
	N0040 4-mm 30 endoscope
	MX2-300 300w light source
	N7000 FOC fiberoptic cable
	PES endoscope system total
	PES Video System
	N2070 Soakable camera
	N2070 OC 30 video coupler
	M547F 10-inch Sony monitor
	PES video system total
	PES system total
	Telescopes and accessories
AT 0233A	4-mm, 30 degree Chakoff telescope, wide angle (autoclavable)
AI 0772 XL	Irrigation/visualization sheath for telescopes AT 0232 and AT 0233
PS 0102	Toledo II sheath for AI 0772
PS 0102 XL	Toledo II sheath for AI 0772 XL
PS 0103	Retraction sheath for AI 0772
PS 0103 XL	Retraction II sheath for AI 0772 XL
LT 0212	10-mm, 0-degree Chakoff telescope
LT 0213	10-mm, 30-degree Chakoff telescope
LT 0215	10-mm, 0-degree Chakoff telescope, short
LT 0216	10-mm, 30-degree Chakoff telescope, short
DS 0102	Toledo dissecting/retraction sheath for use with LT 0212 and LT 0213
PS 1010	Handle for 4-mm telescope
PS 1011	Handle for 10-mm telescope
PS 3062	Endo-Tractor for 10-mm telescope
PS 3063	Endo-Tractor for 4-mm, 30-degree scope
	Instrumentation
PS 0030	Orbital rim dissector, malleable
PS 0031	Microdissector, 3-mm, malleable
PS 0032	Microdissector, 4.5-mm, malleable
PS 0033	Elevator, flat, 6-mm, malleable
PS 0034	Dissector, 10-mm oval, malleable
PS 0035	Frazier suction tube, 4-mm, malleable
PS 0036	Nerve hook, curved, malleable
PS 0037	Periosteal elevator, flat, 13-mm, malleable
PS 0038	Dissector, 6-mm, oval, malleable
PS 0039	Upturned dissector, oval, malleable
PS 0040	Suture passer, malleable
PS 2063	5-mm curved Metzenbaum scissors with cautery, detachable with rotation, 36 cm
PS 2063R	Replacement insert for PS 2063
PS 2075	5-mm hook scissors with cautery, detachable with rotation, 36 cm
PS 2075R	Replacement insert for PS 2075
PS 3061	Soft tissue dissector
PS 3100	Retractable fan retractor
PS 5030	Microjaw curved rotatable Metzenbaum scissors with cautery
PS 5030R	Replacement insert for PS 5030
PS 5030G	Quicksilver axial curved insulated micro-Metzenbaum scissors
PS 5032	Microjaw curved rotatable dissecting forceps with cautery, straight jaws
PS 5032R	Replacement insert for PS 5032
PS 5032G	Quicksilver axial curved insulated microdissecting forceps, straight jaws
PS 5036	Microjaw curved rotatable Kelly dissecting forceps with cautery
PS 5036R	Replacement insert for PS 5036
PS 5038	Curved microspatula with cautery and suction
PS 5039	Same as above, straight
PS 5040	Microjaw curved rotatable Maryland dissecting forceps
PS 5040R	Replacement insert for PS 5040

Continued page 158

TABLE 2. *Continued.*

Storz catalogue number	Description
PS 5040G	Quicksilver axial curved insulated micro-Maryland dissecting forceps
PS 5042	Microjaw curved rotatable grasping forceps with cautery
PS 5042R	Replacement insert for PS 5042
PS 5042G	Quicksilver axial curved insulated micrograsping forceps
PS 5050	Microjaw curved rotatable microhook scissors
PS 5050R	Replacement insert for PS 5050
PS 5050G	Quicksilver axial curved insulated microhook scissors
PS 5080	Long curved spatula with cautery and suction
PS 6011	Handle for dissection, with cautery, all instruments
PS 6012	Handle for grasping, with ratchet, all instruments
PS 6013	Handle, axial
PS 6014	Handle, axial with ratchet
PS 6015	Locking nuts for take apart inst., (pkg of 10)
PS 6050	Knot pusher, curved
PS 6051	Knot pusher, 21 cm
PS 6052	Knot pusher, 36 cm
PS 6053	Knot pusher, 43 cm
PS 7065	5-mm curved Metzenbaum scissors, take apart with cautery, 43-cm length
PS 7065R	Replacement insert for PS 7065
PS 7071	5-mm straight Metzenbaum scissors, take apart with cautery, 43-cm length
PS 7071R	Replacement insert for PS 7071
PS 8000	Monopolar cautery cord
NH 9000	5-mm Chakoff needle holder, long
NH 9001	5-mm Chakoff needle holder, short
NH 9002	5-mm Goldfarb needle holder, 17 cm
NH 9003	5-mm Goldfarb needle holder, 23 cm
NH 9004	5-mm Goldfarb needle holder, 36 cm
AI 0800	Telescoping handle
AI 0809	Hook knife for AI 800
Video and accessories	
VC 0051	Compact video system, immersible with coupler
VC 0052	Office video system with coupler
VC 0053	CCD video camera, hyper HAD CCD, autoexposure greater than 470 lines resolution, with coupler
VC 0062	Three-chip camera, nonimmersible, with coupler
VC 0063	Three-chip camera, immersible, with coupler
PS 706-931	Camera drape, sterile, 7 × 96 in., Box/10
VM 0020	20-in. monitor, high resolution, medical grade
VM 0021	13-in. monitor, high resolution, medical grade
VM 0022	20-in. monitor
VM 0023	13-in. monitor
VA 0094	6-ft. SVHS cable
VA 296	Chakoff, Storz, and Olympus telescope adapter
VA 297	Wolf telescope adapter
VA 298	ACMI telescope adapter
V 300	AC power cord for IEC electric components
Light sources—insufflators	
LS 0011X	300-W xenon light source with turret for ACMI, Wolf, Storz, Olympus
LS 0012	150-W halogen light source
LS 0015	300-W metal halide arc light source
LS 0016	Replacement xenon bulb for LS 0011
LS 0026	Replacement bulb for LS 0012

• Inquire for other light source replacement xenon bulbs
• All xenon light bulbs are guaranteed to last 500 hours, or they will be replaced free of charge

Fiber optic light cables
Specify end fittings (e.g., what brand scope, what brand light source)

FC 0007	5.5-mm, 8-ft. light cable
FC 0008	5.5-mm, 8-ft. light cable, 90° angle, rotatable

• All fiber cables are autoclavable
• Fiber cables can be custom-made to any additional length over 8 ft. at a 10% increase in price. (We recommend a maximum length of 12 ft. for minimum light loss.)

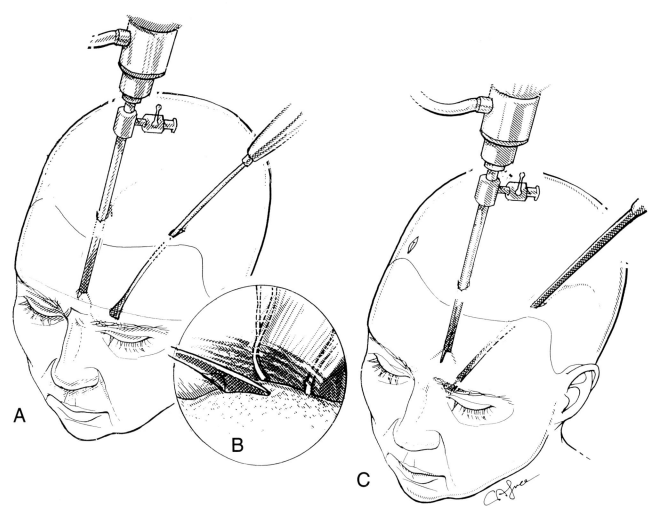

FIG. 21. A: Scope in central part, dissection laterally. **B:** Identification of supraorbital bundles with blunt dissection. **C:** Laser myectomy of corrugator and procerus muscles. (Courtesy of Gregory Chernoff, M.D.)

Observation of the dissection via the camera continues first medially well down onto the root of the nose. The orbital rim is then located, and from medial to lateral, a knuckle-type elevator is utilized to free the periosteum from the orbital rim. This reinforces the fact that blind undermining of the periosteum near the supraorbital rim is a dangerous undertaking.

The laser fiber is then placed through the central incision and used to incise the corrugator and procerus muscles (Table 3). The benefit of a laser for incision is the reduction of postoperative swelling and ecchymosis. The procerus muscle is thin and is located between the corrugator insertions. Its fibers travel vertically upward. The corrugator muscle can be found immediately lateral to the supraperiosteal tunnel over the nose. Its fibers are directed diagonally upward and laterally. Use of the laser to vaporize the muscle fibers allows the supratrochlear nerves to be exposed, as well as preserving the supratrochlear arteries and veins. The supratrochlear nerve can emerge from the same foramen as the supraorbital bundle or can have its own notch or foramen. Muscle that remains posterior and medial to the nerve direction with a slight lateral curvature should be divided. On completion of the central myotomies, the external glabellar folds are then examined. If the muscle was hypertrophied, a 1- to 2-mm patch of Gore-Tex can be placed through the optical cavity into the central region to give more of a bossing effect.

Attention is then directed to the lateral temporal incisions, which are carried through the temporoparietal fascia.

TABLE 3.

Fiber	Fluence
Sharplan 20 Turbinate	10 W superpulse
Surgilase XJ	300 mJ, 8 W
Coherent Ultrapulse	200 mJ, 5 W

This fascia is mobile with movement of the scalp. This dissection is taken down to the deep temporal fascia, which glistens as it lies immediately over the temporalis muscle. The deep temporal fascia does not move when the scalp is retracted upward. By dissecting immediately on top of the deep temporal fascia, the surgeon will keep the facial nerve safe. Posteriorly, this layer is dissected backward over the extent of the temporalis muscle. Medially, under direct vision, the temporal line insertion is dissected using an instrument such as a Sedlot elevator, thereby joining the two dissection planes. Above the innominate fascia, the temporal parietal fat pad containing the facial nerve is visualized. The dissection proceeds downward immediately toward the malar eminence.

If the surgeon wishes to dissect over the zygomatic arch in the subperiosteal plane, a horizontal incision in the superficial layer of deep temporal fascia is made, exposing the superficial fat pad. Basic dissection is carried downward toward the malar eminence, where several perforating branches of the zygomaticotemporal vein can be seen superior to this pad. This will mark the endpoint of the inferior dissection.

Attention is then directed to the subgaleal plane through the central incision. The subgaleal dissection is taken to the posterior occipital incision using a posterior dissector and then carried down posteroinferiorly to the occipital arteries. This ensures absorption of excess tissue and reduction of any potential dog-ear at the point of fixation at the lateral limbal incisions.

Fixation

We use 1.3-mm Synthes Y-shaped microplates and 4-mm screws through the lateral limbal incisions. The region where the bone was previously scored with a laser is identified. The decision as to which hole of the Y-plate to place at this marking depends on how much elevation is required. The straight limb of the Y-plate is pointed inferiorly, with the short limbs placed posteriorly. The straight limb screw is placed first, and this allows an arc of rotation of the Y for a full 180 degrees. The arc of pull of the lateral brow is then determined, and this determines the placement of the remaining two screws for the Y-plate (Fig. 22A–C).

With an assistant holding the posteriorly displaced scalp at the appropriate vector and level, a permanent suture of 2-0 Ethibond is placed through the periosteum and under the Y of the plate. The incisions are then closed in a layered fashion, and a head dressing is applied.

Complications

The most frequent complications seen in this procedure include ecchymosis, seroma, numbness, paresis, stitch abscess, neuropraxia of the facial nerve, incisional alopecia, failure to correct brow ptosis, and relapse of brow ptosis.

To date, no permanent paralysis of the temporal branch of the facial nerve has been reported in the literature.

Most authors agree that there seems to be a reduced incidence in severity of complications with the endoscopic approach compared with large-incisional procedures. The greatest advantages include avoidance of lifting hair-bearing scalp and avoidance of injury to the supraorbital nerve. Patient acceptance of the endoscopic forehead lift also far exceeds that for coronal brow lifts, which were previously performed.

Endoscopic Midfacelift

Patient Selection

The endoscopic midfacelift procedure is selected when lifting of the inferior and lateral periorbital soft tissues is desired. This is performed by repositioning the malar and nasal jugal fat pads. Another indication for this procedure is the presence of deep nasolabial folds and laxity of the orbicularis muscle, yielding excessive scleral show.

The endoscopic midfacelift can be classified proportionally to the level of dissection. These include a suborbicularis-suprazygomatic dissection (commonly referred to as the malar pad lift), a subperiosteal dissection, or a subcutaneous dissection.

Subperiosteal Midfacelift

A subperiosteal midfacelift is indicated in very thin, elderly patients with hypoplastic malar fat pads and severe nasolabial folds requiring wide undermining. The main advantage of an endoscopic approach is the ability to lift the midface without the need for a preauricular incision. A drawback of this approach is the significant postoperative edema that may last months. The incisions utilized include two temporal incisions, one superior and close to the temporal line and one inferior, close, and posterior to the region of the side burn. A lower blepharoplasty incision can be utilized, as well as an incision through a natural crease in the region of the crow's-feet. A Caldwell-Luc incision can be added to elevate the periosteum on the maxilla and malar area in a retrograde fashion. The dissection is performed under the periosteum on the lateral orbital rim, zygomatic arch, and maxilla inferiorly. The periosteum is detached from its inferior attachment at the level of the zygomatic arch and maxilla. Suspension sutures of 4-0 clear Prolene are placed at the level of the suborbicularis fat pad or just inferior to it. Suspension sutures in the temporal incisions will not produce significant elevation of the midface due to the large amount of tissue detachment and the differing plane of dissection in relation to the temporal region.

The main advantage of the endoscopic subperiosteal midfacelift is the ability to lift the midface without the need for a preauricular incision. The ability to excise lower lid

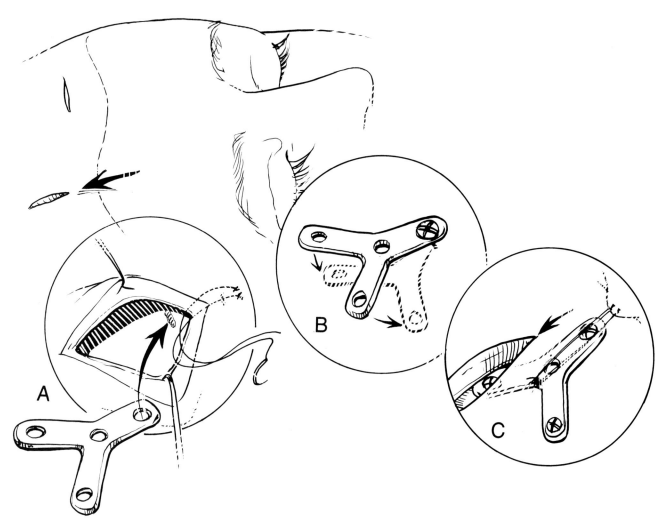

FIG. 22. Fixation: **A:** Titanium Y-plate in limbus-level incision. **B:** Arc of rotation is variable depending on first-stem fixation. Rotation is proportional to the vector of the desired elevation. **C:** Full-thickness suture "O Ticron" suspends around the apex of the plate. (Courtesy of Gregory Chernoff, M.D.)

skin with less risk of ectropion due to the motion obtained in the malar area is also an advantage. Repositioning of the midface soft tissue in the subperiosteal plane allows the zygomaticus major and minor muscles to be lifted in a superolateral direction. This leads inevitably to an upturning of the commissures of the mouth. The subperiosteal approach has been criticized for its inability to improve the nasolabial fold to any extent. This is because there is little change in the position of the malar pad with respect to the underlying facial muscles. The nasolabial fold is formed by fascial fibers connecting the dermis in the underlying superficial muscles of facial expression. Over time, rotation of the malar fat pad in a medial and inferior direction causes further deepening of the fold.

This region of the zygomatic arch is the danger area with respect to the frontal branch of the facial nerve. The overlying periosteum of the zygomatic arch is the only pro-

tection of the nerve at this level. Careful attention to detail must be observed to avoid inadvertent injury to the nerve.

Supraperiosteal Midfacelift (Malar Pad Lift)

The supraperiosteal midfacelift or malar pad lift is indicated in patients requiring midfacelift to treat moderate to deep nasolabial folds and improve sagginess in the malar orbital area. As with all midface approaches, this can be performed in conjunction with an endoscopic brow lift or separately utilizing the aforementioned temporal incisions. A preauricular rhytidectomy incision will not be required in either of these scenarios. The endoscopic malar pad lift can also be performed during a rhytidectomy with or without a brow plasty to provide midface rejuvenation in place of a deep-plane or composite lift. If this technique is used in conjunction with a rhytidectomy, the lateral orbital incision is not required. The net effect of the endoscopic malar pad lift is to reposition the fibrofatty tissue in a posterosuperior vector lateral to the nasolabial fold. This yields an improvement in the depth of the nasolabial fold, as well as in the contour of the malar area. Caution must be utilized with the supraperiosteal approach in patients who are ectomorphic in the malar region, as lifting this area with suture fixation can result in skin dimpling.

Through the lower blepharoplasty incision or crow's-feet incision, dissection is carried down through the orbicularis muscle. The orbicularis muscle overlies the zygomaticus major muscle, and the buccal branch of the facial nerve enters underneath the zygomaticus major muscle. As the orbicularis is retracted superiorly, dissection is carried out underneath the muscle until the head of the zygomaticus major muscle is identified at its attachment to the malar eminence. Caution is utilized to stay superficial to the fascial layer investing the zygomaticus. The head is dissected to the point that a finger can be inserted. A dissection pocket is created between the underlying zygomaticus muscle and the overlying fascia, fat, and skin. The direction of the dissection is parallel to the zygomaticus toward the labial commissure.

The suborbicularis fat pad and the malar fat pad are then suspended in a posterior and vertical direction with 2-0 PDS sutures to the deep temporal fascia or infrazygomatic fascia. This then effectively improves midface ptosis of these structures. Patients with excess skin require removal at the temporal incision or at the preauricular site.

Subcutaneous Midfacelift

This technique is employed in patients with moderate midface ptosis and early jowling; it is usually performed in conjunction with the malar pad lift. Two incisions are placed in the preauricular area, measuring 2 cm in length. Subcutaneous undermining is performed. Two oblique incisions are made in the SMAS. The superior SMAS flap is developed on top of the zygomatic arch, measuring 1 cm in width, and extends to the origin of the zygomaticus major muscle. A lower SMAS flap is developed toward the labial commissure. On elevation of these SMAS flaps, excess is then excised and 2-0 PDS sutures are placed, permitting elevation and rotation of the SMAS in an upward posterior direction with attachment in the preauricular region. Rarely does skin have to be excised.

Endoscopic Neck Lift

As age increases and gravitational forces cause tissues to head in a southerly direction, so can endoscopic procedures. While this continues to be the realm of rhytidectomy, submental lipectomy, and platysmal plication, use of an endoscopic approach in patients requiring plastysmaplasty is increasing in popularity. This provides the opportunity to diminish the size of the incision used in typical face and neck lifts. In the absence of platysmal bands greater than 1 cm deep, the submental incision can be omitted, and the procedure performed through two postauricular incisions measuring 2 cm in length. This approach should not be used in patients who have isolated lipodystrophies of the submental region with elastic skin, who would benefit from liposuction alone. The procedure is mainly indicated when improvement in submental fullness is desired and when suture plication of the submental bands alone does not fully resolve the fullness. The procedure permits an upward and posterior traction sling to be placed on the platysma, as described by Giampapa and modified by Keller.

With a patient that has some subcutaneous fat and platysmal banding, the procedure is commenced by a 1-cm submental incision, with subsequent liposculpture in the region. Postauricular incisions are then fashioned, and the endoscope is inserted, with subcutaneous elevation utilizing the laser fiber. The tunnels are connected, and the platysma muscle is identified. A 2-0 PDS suture is placed through the submental incision in a horizontal mattress fashion through one of the platysmal bands. It is then passed through the subcutaneous plane under endoscopic vision to the opposite mastoid. A vertical mattress suture is placed through the opposite platysmal band and extended to the opposing mastoid. The sutures are then placed through the mastoid processes. If additional lower plication of the platysma is required, this is performed through the submental incision.

Rarely does this postauricular incision have to be extended with skin excision.

Summary

Endoscope-assisted surgical approaches to the upper one-third and lower one-third of the face continue to be refined. Through this process, tighter indications and limitations are being defined. This has given the aesthetic surgeon the ability to conservatively create improvements in these facial regions through smaller incisions. With smaller access ports, the surgeon must possess much clearer knowledge of the anatomy of the operated region to avoid damage to important structures. With these modified approaches, earlier intervention to the aging process is achievable for patients seeking aesthetic change before gravitational forces have significant effects.

The advent of laser fibers allowing dissection with improved hemostasis has further advanced the field of endoscopic minimally invasive surgery. While this is an exciting field, patient safety should never be compromised, and time-tested techniques should continue to be respected and offered to patients who benefit from them to a greater degree.

CHAPTER 14

Adjunctive Techniques

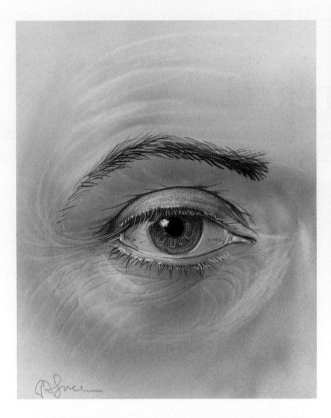

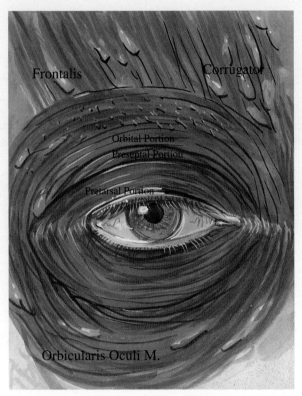

Frontalis

Corrugator

Orbital Portion

Preseptal Portion

Pretarsal Portion

Orbicularis Oculi M.

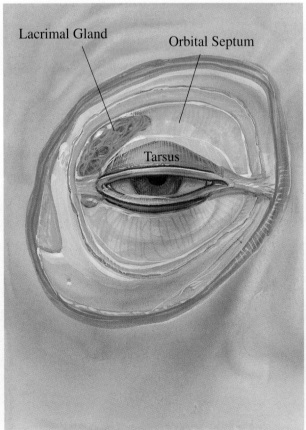

Lacrimal Gland

Orbital Septum

Tarsus

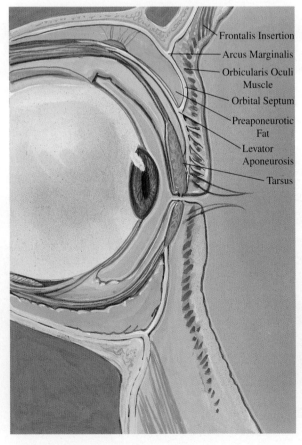

Frontalis Insertion

Arcus Marginalis

Orbicularis Oculi
Muscle

Orbital Septum

Preaponeurotic
Fat

Levator
Aponeurosis

Tarsus

Since the first edition of this volume, the quality of the final result following eyelid and facial rejuvenation has seen further improvement. Surface irregularities and residual static rhytids following blepharoplasty and browplasty can largely be ablated with laser resurfacing. Facial contour redundancy secondary to skin flaccidity can also be markedly improved with laser resurfacing. Any residual dynamic rhytids and surface depressions can be addressed with volume augmentation (Table 1), chemodenervation, and adjunctive facial surgical techniques (see Chapter 13). These include inferior and superior sulcus deformities, glabellar furrows, deeper crow's-feet, and laugh lines.

VOLUME-AUGMENTATION TECHNIQUES

Bovine Collagen

Bovine collagen injections have yielded transient reduction in facial rhytids. The drawbacks of this technique have been rapid recurrence of rhytids (3 months or less in most patients), a low but significant incidence of postinjection inflammatory response with subsequent subdermal fibrosis in some patients, and intimations of a relationship between bovine collagen injection and autoimmune disease. In addition, repeated injections do not necessarily last longer. Before facial rhytid augmentation is performed, an intradermal test dose of 0.1 mL is given in the retroauricular area or the volar surface of the forearm. During the following 4 weeks, any inflammatory signs are noted as an indication of allergy. Bovine collagen is supplied in three forms: Zyderm I, Zyderm II, and Zyplast (Collagen Corporation, Calif).

Zyderm I

This highly purified bovine collagen derivative is used for filling fine wrinkles. Zyderm I is prepackaged in 0.5- and 1-mL syringes with 27-gauge needles. Each syringe contains saline, lidocaine, and 30% to 35% collagen. Each implant is delivered in a gel that becomes a soft tissue mass within 3 to 4 days after injection. Four weeks after test-site injection, the injections are given intradermally in the area of depression and overcorrected by approximately 60% to 100%. Within 48 hours, the lidocaine and saline will have dispersed. This bioimplant, however, is not permanent, and most patients require repeat injections within 3 months or less.

Zyderm II

Zyderm II is injected more deeply into the epidermis. Overcorrection is not recommended, and the area of implantation must be massaged at the time of injection until the desired effect is achieved. It is resorbed more slowly than is Zyderm I. It is used to augment deeper facial furrows (glabellar, forehead, nasolabial).

Zyplast

Zyplast also is resorbed more slowly than is Zyderm I. It is applied in the same manner and locations as Zyderm II, and many physicians find it more reliable than Zyderm II.

Autogenous Collagen

Autogenous collagen may yield increased longevity. Collagenesis (Acton, Mass) isolates collagen from resected skin. Following a rhytidectomy, there is enough resected skin to provide a sufficient amount of autogenous collagen. However, eyelid skin resections in blepharoplasty will only yield a small amount of injectable material, which might not be adequate to correct the objectionable deformity. Subsequent injections will require additional harvesting of tissue to be processed.

Isolagen (Paramus, NJ) uses a small punch biopsy to grow autogenous fibroblasts and collagen. This technique perhaps holds the potential for a long lasting correction. The initial

TABLE 1. *Volume-augmentation techniques*

	Hyaluronic acid gel[a]	Bovine collagen	Autogenous cell culture (Isolagen)	Autogenous reprocessed (Collagenesis)	Microlipoinjection
Injected via 30-gauge needle	Yes	Yes	Yes	Yes	No
Tissue harvesting	No	No	Yes	Yes	Yes
Additional harvesting for repeat injections	No	No	No	Yes	On occasion
Increased longevity with repeated injections	No	No	Yes	Variable	Variable

[a] Not available in the United States.

cell culture is frozen and stored and can be reutilized whenever additional material is necessary; this will not require any additional donor material. However, the cells of very old patients or patients with severe actinic damage may not grow sufficiently to supply enough cell volume for correction of the defects. The technique reportedly works well when combined with laser facial resurfacing. The biopsy is taken at the time of resurfacing. About 1.5 mL of cell culture will be available for injection in 4 to 5 weeks. The facial dermis at that stage of healing and collagenogenesis is apparently receptive to the implantation of the new fibroblasts. There is about 10% to 15% residual filling effect 3 months following the first injection, 30% to 50% following the second injection, and 70% to 80% following the third injection. Most patients require two to three injections for an effect that will last longer than 6 months.

Microlipoinjection

Fat cells harvested by liposuction have been injected into facial rhytids with some success (see Chapter 13).

Hyaluronic Acid Gel

Hyaluronic acid gel [e.g., Hylaform (Biomatrix, Saint Tropez, France), Restylane (Q Med, Uppsala, Sweden)] is not yet available for use in the United States, although it has been approved for use in Europe and South America.

It is a naturally occurring mucopolysaccharide, not a protein, so it will not induce a foreign body reaction when it is injected. It is an altered form of Healon (Pharmacia, Kalamazoo, MI), which has been used intraocularly during cataract surgery for almost 20 years. It can be injected via a 30-gauge needle to augment static rhytids with great accuracy. The consistency of the gel makes it easy to use and to fill deformities with precision. After 1 year, 60% remains. As it is absorbed, its great affinity for water allows it to maintain its volume (Figs. 1A,B, 2A–C). A thicker version (not yet available) will require a 25-gauge needle for injection, but it may last 2 to 3 years.

DERMABRASION

Since the advent of laser resurfacing, dermabrasion has become largely obsolete. It is less effective and less easily controlled and has a higher incidence of dyspigmentation and scarring. Because facial skin is 25 times thicker than eyelid skin, cautious use of dermabrasion can flatten raised defects in the facial skin. However, we have seen overuse of this technique that has resulted in dermal thinning and cicatrization (particularly in the upper lip area).

Cautious use of dermabrasion on facial skin removes keratinized epithelium, superficial dermis, and raised defects of the skin surface, allowing reepithelialization of this surface. It will not remove wrinkles and is not effective in correcting depressed areas. It is not recommended for use

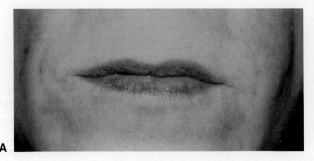
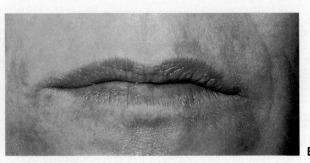

FIG. 1. A: This 38-year-old woman with narrow lips desired augmentation. **B:** Following two 0.8-mL syringes of hyaluronic acid gel, adequate augmentation is noted.

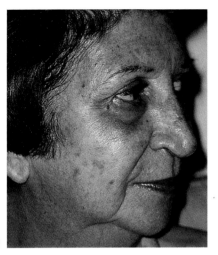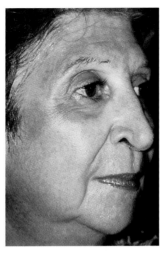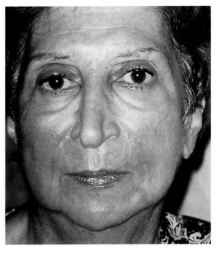

A, B

FIG. 2. A: This 67-year-old woman had full superior sulci, lower lid prolapsed fat, and moderate facial dyspigmentation with rhytidosis. **B:** Her appearance improved following internal transblepharoplasty brow contouring and suspension with full-face CO_2 laser resurfacing. **C:** Three months later hyaluronic acid gel was used to fill in and soften her nasolabial folds.

on the eyelids. Eyelid skin is exceptionally thin and movable, technically difficult to dermabrade, and easily gouged and abraded too deeply.

CHEMICAL PEELS

Chemical peels can prepare patients for laser facial resurfacing and can complement carbon dioxide (CO_2) laser rejuvenation, depending on the agent used. In this environment, there are no indications for phenol peels. Resurfacing with the CO_2 laser or erbium:yttrium-aluminum-garnet (Er:YAG) laser permits greater control, and in appropriately selected and prepared patients, the risk of dyspigmentation is minimized. Whereas the long-term effects of phenol peels make subsequent facial surgery difficult, laser resurfacing facilitates and potentiates subsequent cosmetic facial procedures.

Trichloroacetic acid (TCA) 25% or 35% can be used to blend and feather the neck, which cannot at this time be effectively treated with the CO_2 or Er:YAG lasers.

Alpha-hydroxy acids (AHAs) are a standard part of a maintenance regimen, and they may have some role in the preparation of the patient for laser facial rejuvenation. They may also be helpful in the late-postoperative phase in more quickly reducing transient hyperpigmentation.

BOTOX

Originally used in the treatment of incapacitating blepharospasm over 15 years ago, botulinum toxin type A purified neurotoxin complex (Botox) is an effective transient remedy for dynamic facial rhytids (Fig. 3A–C). It chemically denervates the myoneurojunction. We have found it

particularly useful in flattening glabellar furrows, transverse forehead creases, and periocular rhytids and crow's-feet. It enhances the effect of laser resurfacing in these areas. Because it takes 3 to 5 days to have an effect, we prefer to inject it at least 1 week before laser resurfacing or immediately following laser resurfacing. Its effect can last 3 to 6 months following the first injections. When followed by laser resurfacing, it can last longer. Subsequent administrations of Botox can often be delayed 8 to 10 months.

Botox is supplied freeze-dried in 100-U bottles. Before being used, it must be thawed and diluted with nonbacteriostatic sterile saline. For ease of administration, it can be diluted into various strengths. We have found it convenient to dilute it in 5-mL aliquots (20 U/mL) and to inject it in 0.1-mL aliquots. Although electromyography can be used for exact placement of the injections, this is usually not necessary (Fig. 4). We have found that subcutaneous rather than intramuscular injections lessen the chance of hematoma formation and are equally effective. Injections are placed on either side of the rhytid and approximate the corrugator and procerus muscle insertions. About 20 U is used in the glabella and 40 U in the forehead. We use between 10 to 15 U for crow's-feet (each side). Once mixed, Botox is best used within the next 1 to 2 hours.

SOLID SYNTHETIC IMPLANTS

Various one-piece implants have been used to augment the periocular facial contour, to fill in depressions of the medial eyelid (tear trough), or to build up the malar eminence. Some of the materials used include polymethyl methacrylate, hydroxyapatite, and expanded polytetrafluo-

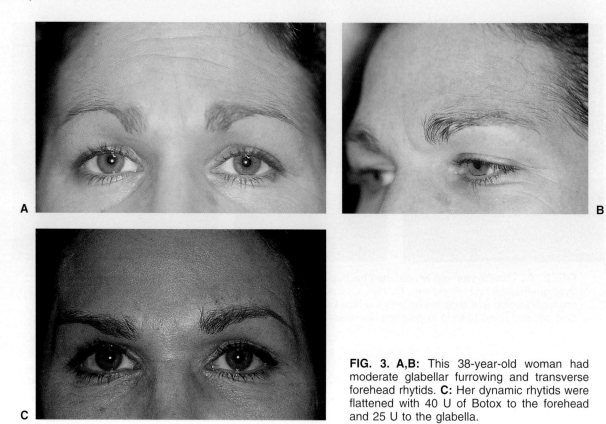

FIG. 3. A,B: This 38-year-old woman had moderate glabellar furrowing and transverse forehead rhytids. **C:** Her dynamic rhytids were flattened with 40 U of Botox to the forehead and 25 U to the glabella.

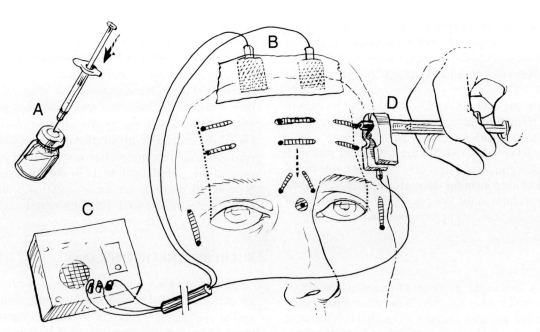

FIG. 4. Although electromyography was initially used to confirm the placement of Botox injections, we no longer find this necessary. Supplied freeze-dried in 100-U bottles, it is reconstituted in 5 mL to 10 mL of saline.

roethylene. These implants may be inserted via transconjunctival or intraoral techniques.

TOPICAL AGENTS

Tretinoin (Retinoic Acid)

Nightly applications of tretinoin (Retin-A) 0.1% mixed 1:3 with a noncomedogenic emollient cream has been found to provide definite reversal of photodamaged skin. The area to be treated is washed and then thoroughly dried. A small amount of the tretinoin preparation is applied into the undesired wrinkles with a toothpick and then rubbed superficially into the area. After as short a time as several weeks, some improvement of fine wrinkling and hyperpigmentation has been described. With longer application, improvement in coarse wrinkling has been noted. Many patients using this regimen experience an initial prolonged erythema that lasts weeks to months; some experience a recurrent dermatitis. The erythema and scaly dermatitis can be lessened with concomitant applications of lubricants or topical steroid preparations. Prolonged application of tretinoin will decrease cutaneous melanin and increase cutaneous photosensitivity. Patients applying this preparation must be instructed to wear a sun block.

Alpha-hydroxy Acid

Tretinoin and AHAs have been incorporated into the regimen of many physicians preparing their patients for laser resurfacing. Combining these agents with hydroquinone and/or kojic acid minimizes postinflammatory hyperpigmentation and can also enhance reepithelialization.

Topical Vitamin C

Recognized as a powerful antioxidant, topical preparations containing Vitamin C are an effective agent in reducing fine rhytids and in enhancing healing following laser resurfacing (when the acute inflammatory phase has passed).

DECREASING SUPERIOR ORBITAL RIM PROMINENCE: BURRING DOWN ORBITAL RIMS

Prominent superior orbital rims can be thinned by resecting the brow fat pocket and orbicularis muscle overlying the superior orbital rim. But in extreme cases, burring down the orbital rim may be considered.

Patients with excessive prominence of the superior orbital rim, casting the upper lid and superior sulcus into dark shadows and creating a concave contour deformity most obvious just inferior to the orbital rim, may be pleased with the results of shaving off or burring away the anterior aspect of the superior orbital rim. The rims may be exposed via superior blepharoplasty incisions. A high-speed air drill

can be used to burr down the bone. Extreme care must be used to provide a smooth bony surface and to avoid the neurovascular bundles, which must be retracted. The burred down orbital rims may be covered with an absorbable gelatin sponge (e.g., Gelfoam) to provide a smooth contour.

CORRECTING INFERIOR ORBITAL CONTOUR IRREGULARITIES

Fat Pedicle Flap Transposition

Concave deformities of the inferior orbit can be softened by transposing fat pedicle flaps via a transconjunctival or transcutaneous approach. While still attached to a vascular pedicle, orbital fat can be mobilized and shifted to area to be augmented.

Microlipoinjection

See ''Autologous Microlipoaugmentation (Fat Transfers),'' Chapter 13.

Malar and Tear-trough Implants

Hypotrophic malar eminence and medial orbital depressions can be augmented with premolded methyl methacrylate implants applied via intraoral or transconjunctival approaches.

RHYTIDECTOMY

Laser eyelid and facial rejuvenation has not completely eliminated the need for rhytidectomy in some patients. Marked facial skin and muscle redundancy will require this procedure. Residual redundancies following full-face resurfacing will also require rhytidectomy. Conversely, patients who have had a well executed rhytidectomy may still have a facial skin patina that will benefit from full-face laser resurfacing. Following a rhytidectomy, a patient should wait at least 3 months before undergoing full-face resurfacing. The converse is true as well: A patient should wait at least 3 months following full-face resurfacing before undergoing a rhytidectomy.

The problem of generalized facial laxity should be anticipated preoperatively, and a rhytidectomy or full-face resurfacing should be recommended and performed at the time of the blepharoplasty. Rhytidectomy provides periocular structural support inferiorly and is analogous to bicoronal scalp resections for brow and upper lid support. It supports the cheek and malar complex and removes weight and drag from the lower lids.

RADIOSURGICAL REMOVAL OF BENIGN FACIAL AND EYELID LESIONS

The use of fine-wire radiosurgical electrodes (Ellman International, Hewlett, NY) is a convenient, safe, and effective technique for removing flat and/or elevated lesions of the face and eyelids. Operating at a frequency of 3.8 megahertz (MHz), it generates little lateral heat spread. It is not a cautery, and uses an antenna, not a grounding pad.

Using a topical anesthetic paste containing lidocaine 2.5% and prilocaine 2.5% (EMLA) and loop electrodes of varying sizes, these lesions can be removed in the operating room or in the examining room with exquisite accuracy (Fig. 5).

TREATMENT OF FACIAL LESIONS AND VASCULAR, TELANGIECTATIC, AND PIGMENTED LESIONS

The following alternative means are now available to treat facial lesions that were previously not amenable to resection. In most instances, local anesthesia is not required.

Argon Laser

The argon laser delivers blue-green light (488 to 514 nm) and up to 30 W. It can be used without anesthetic to treat port-wine stains and hemangiomas.

Tunable Dye Laser

This laser uses yellow light (400 to 800 nm) and up to 5 W can be delivered. When used at 585 nm, it can be used for port-wine stains and telangiectases.

Copper Vapor Laser

This laser operates at 578 nm and can be used as a treatment for port-wine stains.

KTP Laser

The KTP laser, a frequency-doubled neodymium: yttrium-aluminum-garnet (Nd:YAG) laser, delivers green light at 532 nm. It is comparable to the argon laser in its usefulness for treating vascular lesions. Up to 20 W can be delivered.

Laser Hair Removal

We offer our patients who will undergo full-face resurfacing laser hair removal (with the long-pulse Alexandrite or the Q-Switched YAG laser) prior to the resurfacing. It is particularly useful in men because they will not be able to shave for the next 3 to 4 weeks.

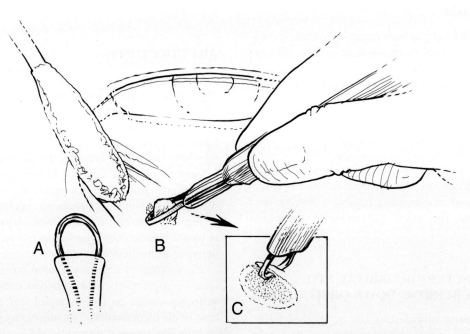

FIG. 5. A radiosurgical loop electrode can accurately shave raised and flat benign facial lesions.

CHAPTER 15

Perioperative Care of Eyelid and Facial Rejuvenation Patients

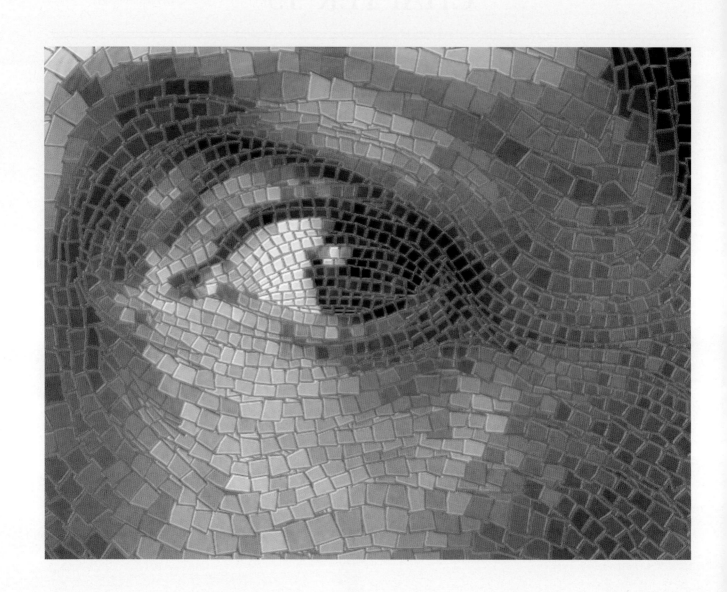

Perioperative care of patients who have had resurfacing is critical. It will make the difference between a successful result and a less satisfactory one. Close monitoring after resurfacing will prevent possible complications that may compromise the results of treatment. In addition, these patients need psychologic, as well as physical support. When the results are maximized, they are impressive, but this requires time and effort from the surgeon and his or her staff.

Preoperatively, patients must be impressed with the need to follow instructions meticulously. They should be aware of the possibility of transient postinflammatory hyperpigmentation. They should understand the necessity of prophylactic antiherpetic and antibacterial medication. They must understand that during the healing phase following resurfacing, their skin will be exceptionally sensitive, and they should only use products that their surgeon approves. The use of anything else can cause a serious reaction. For instance, it may be a patient's perception that aloe vera is soothing and can aid healing. Unfortunately, aloe vera can also be a potent sensitizing agent and cannot be used postoperatively.

Because the perfect postoperative regimen does not exist, our management of these patients is in a constant state of evolution with frequent modifications and improvements.

PREOPERATIVE REGIMEN

While it has become apparent that topical bleaching agents, alpha-hydroxy acids (AHAs), and tretinoin (Retin-A) used preoperatively may not affect the final result, a basic cleansing protocol followed by nourishment and hydration of the skin is given, as well as systemic prophylaxis (Table 1). We still use preoperative bleaching and AHA agents in patients with marked pigment irregularities or thick skin (stratum corneum). Private-label products are available, but some are of poor quality and many are simply relabeled old products. We prefer to have our own products privately compounded by a cosmetic chemist, and in this

manner we can be assured of the quality and contents of what our patients use. We give our patients a preoperative check list (Table 2).

IMMEDIATE POSTOPERATIVE TREATMENT

For resurfaced patients, we need to choose what kind of dressings to use immediately after the procedure. Dressings can be open or closed. Open dressings represent the application of ointments, without the actual dressing. We have found that closed dressings promote a moist healing environment that increases the level of comfort, reduces pruritus, produces less erythema, and decreases the exudative phase of wound healing.

The following are some of the closed dressings that are available:

- Flexzan (Dow Hickam Pharmaceuticals, Inc., Sugar Land, TX) is a polyurethane dressing, bilayered, with an adhesive side. It is semiocclusive (has small pores), which allows vapor and some exudation to be released from the wound. It is opaque and very often needs to be replaced in the office during the critical reepithelialization phase.
- N-Terface (Winfield Laboratories) is a mesh dressing that consists of a fine, high-density polyethylene sheeting with some absorptive effect.

TABLE 1. *Preoperative prophylaxis*

Two days preop
  Mupirocin (Bactroban) intranasally twice daily.
  Lysine 500 mg twice daily
One day preop
  Mupirocin intranasally b.i.d.
  Cephalosporin (e.g., Keflex) 250 mg p.o. b.i.d.[a]
  Acyclovir (Zovirax) 400 mg t.i.d.,[a] or famciclovir (Famvir) 250 mg* daily,[a] or valacyclovir (Valtrex) 500 mg b.i.d.[a]
  Lysine 500 mg b.i.d.[a]

[a] Continued until reepithelialization is complete.

173

TABLE 2. *Laser preop home care instructions*

Prior to laser surgery

The following regimen is recommended to ensure the best result from your laser resurfacing. It is designed to remove the upper layers of skin to get a more even result. The regimen will also aid in the healing process and prevent any problems with pigmentation. The vitamins support the healing process internally, while the creams support the process externally. It is extremely important to follow your individualized regimen carefully to optimize your final result.

AM
1. Preop cleanser ( )
2. Fade cream 4% ( )
3. Eye gel ( )
4. Day lotion with SPF-15 ( )
5. Glycolic acid product ( )

PM
1. Preop cleanser ( )
2. Fade cream 4% ( )
3. Eye gel ( )
4. Glycolic acid product ( )
5. Night cream ( )

One day prior to laser surgery
1. Take the following antiviral agent
    ( ) Famvir   125 mg twice a day
    ( ) Zovirax   400 mg three times a day
    ( ) Valtrex   500 mg twice a day
    ( ) Lysine   500 mg twice a day
2. Keflex 250 mg (antibiotic) twice a day
3. Bactroban (ointment) intranasally
4. Wash hair and face with Phisohex
5. Lymphatic drainage massage ( ) Yes ( ) No

Preop Program

Should be started as soon as you know you'll have the procedure done

Topical program

Pre-op cleanser: Nondetergent cleanser that not only cleanses skin of impurities but also moisturizes and softens skin. It preserves the natural lipid barrier on the skin surface. It should be used in the morning and at night.
Remove makeup, mascara, and debris with a small amount of the cleanser on a cotton pad or soft wash cloth; then rinse with tap water. There will be a film on the skin that will treat and nourish it at the same time.

Fade cream 2% or 4%: It is designed to lighten the area to be treated with the laser and prevent hyperpigmentation after laser resurfacing.
Glycolic acid gel or lotion: To be used after facial cleansing twice daily.
Eye gel: To be applied around eyes, morning and night. This has active ingredients that reduce subcutaneous fat around the eyes and at the same time stimulate deeper layers of skin to produce more collagen and elastin.
Day lotion with SPF-15: Use of this lotion is easy and more effective after the skin has been cleansed with the preop cleanser. The antioxidants and all active nutrients from this lotion quickly penetrate the skin to protect it. A SPF-15 was added to this formula for your comfort and protection. (You do not need to use another sun protector, unless you are using another moisturizer and hydrating cream without SPF.)
Re-apply the day lotion with SPF 15 if you are outdoors. The use of hats and sunglasses is highly recommended. You may use makeup now, after applying the day lotion.
Night cream: This is a reconstructive cream, enriched with high levels of vitamin A, vitamin E, and other immune-stimulants and antioxidants. This is carefully designed to the circadian rhythm of the body, where restoration occurs at night.

Systemic program

Antiviral: The need will be specified by your physician. To be started 1 day before the procedure.
Lysine: 1,000 mg/day (500 mg twice a day)
Antibiotic: To be started the day before surgery by your physician, if you are having full-face resurfacing only.
Vitamins and internal supplements: These supplements help prepare the skin for surgery and help the repair process after surgery. After surgical recovery is complete, their continued, long-term use continues to protect skin and reverse environmental hazards, especially skin cancer and aging.
After continued use, the skin will become more elastic, and the color will assume an even and healthy uniformity. Blemishes and brown spots will disappear, and the skin will become softer and smoother.
Additional protective ingredients have been added to control the free radicals in the skin and the body: These are essential to speed up the repair process. Proteolytic enzymes are included to reduce puffiness and inflammation after surgery.

- Second Skin is a dressing classified as a hydrogel (plastic sheeting composed of 96% water and 4% polyethylene mesh). It has to be changed on a daily basis, and patients find that it is not too practical, since there are too many steps involved in such a procedure.
- Silon-TRS (Bio Med Sciences, Inc.), classified as a polymer, is a thin sheeting of silicone polymers. It allows oxygen and moist vapor to exude and protects the wound from external agents.

In our practice, we choose to use Flexzan and Silon-TRS. They both are relatively easy to apply (Flexzan is more time-consuming) and very often has to be replaced in the office when displaced during the critical healing phase. Additional ointment is required around eyes, mouth, tip of the nose, and contour of the face. Rarely do patients require anything more potent than acetaminophen for discomfort.

POSTOPERATIVE CARE: DAYS 1 TO 7

Tables 3 and 4 summarize the postoperative care regimens.

TABLE 3. *Postoperative days 1–7*

Continue Mupirocin (Bactroban) intranasally t.i.d.
Continue antibiotic
Continue antiviral
To prevent secondary infection, wash the exposed areas twice or three times a day with a postop nonirritating dilute germicidal cleanser (postop cleanser) or a solution of acetic acid 10% diluted in 1L of water, depending on the amount of oozing and crusting.

If the semiocclusive dressings are kept in place, patients will have a relatively good level of comfort. They have to supplement the nonocclusive areas with proper emollients, and great attention should be given to the hygiene of exposed areas to prevent crusting formation. We instruct our patients to keep their head elevated and to keep a clean towel around the neck to collect any exudation.

The crusting should be gently but effectively cleansed with a soft cloth soaked with a solution of acetic acid 10% (one tablespoon diluted in 1 L of water) or our Postlaser cleanser (Total Rejuvenation Systems, New York, NY).

At all times, patients should have a humidifier next to their face, and during the winter the heating vent should be kept off in their room.

After the first week, patients should be checked at least on a weekly basis to make sure that the healing is taking its course and to adjust their daily routine of systemic medication and topical applications. The physiologic reassurance is fundamental from the surgeon, as well as the whole office staff. Make yourself and your staff available to your patients!

After the tenth day, systemic medication is discontinued, and patients should continue the cleansing–hydrating routine.

In general, around the second week in humid climates and the third week in dry locations, patients should be introduced to camouflage makeup, which not only allows them to return to their activities but also protects their extrasensitive skin against external agents, especially the sun.

Patients should be advised (according to their skin color and classification) about the possibilities of secondary and temporary hyperpigmentation changes. In our experience, such changes are reversible and require proper care. With darker skin, there is also the possibility of permanent hypopigmentation.

We like to emphasize that in our vast experience with multiethnic skin types, we have never had hypopigmentation. We believe that our success is due to being conservative with the delivery of laser energy and being careful with the management of patients.

Cosmetic surgeons should make it clear to their patients that the erythema that occurs after laser resurfacing (either carbon dioxide or erbium) are temporary and represent a response of the body that will promote a therapeutic effect—more collagen formation.

TABLE 4. *Postoperative regimens*

Postresurfacing program

Starting with good skin from our preop program, we are now facing a 6–7-day critical postop period.

- Continue with the vitamins and internal supplements.
- Keep your head elevated on a pillow; change pillow on daily basis or a few times a day if necessary.

Initial days postop

Mask: It is a unique, comfortable, and effective existing system to promote tissue healing and absorb blood and serum. It provides a germ-free covering and a cooling moist compress that can last up to 5 days. You may need to change your mask during this 5-day period. Your physician will discuss the need with you.

Dressing: You may be using a *closed dressing* on the resurfaced area or some *heavy emollient*. The purpose of either one is the same as the mask: to promote quicker and more comfortable healing. You may need to change the dressing during those initial 5–7 days. You will be given instructions by your doctor.

Postlaser cleanser: This germicidal cleanser is used directly on skin when oil- and emulsion-based cleansers should be avoided. It can be used in between the applications of the healing mask or dressings, or when the skin is not occluded. Because of its germicidal properties, it cleanses and purifies raw skin when it is in its most vulnerable condition.

After mask or dressing removal

When the mask or dressings are removed, wash the skin with *Postlaser cleanser* twice a day.

Apply *Postlaser balm* in *generous* amounts, as many times as necessary during the day and night.

The skin may be red, itch, and feel dry. The constant use of the postlaser balm, with all its nutrients and healing factors, will normalize the skin.

- DON'T USE GAUZE: Use a very soft cloth, soaked with water, to help the cleansing.
- DON'T PULL ANY EXISTING CRUST: Let it fall off by itself!

Second or third week after resurfacing

You may use camouflage makeup to cover up any areas where you might have discoloration.

- You should not bleach or dye the hair for 30 days following the procedure.
- You should not wax, have electrolysis, chemical hair removal, or laser hair removal on the face for at least 30 days following the procedure.

Postop instructions for CO_2 resurfaced and eyelid surgery patients

Ice packs: Keep ice packs or an ice mask on the surgical area, if you had eyelid surgery, for at least the first 48 hours. If you are taking any medication, you may reinstate it.

Dressings: If you have dressings, they should be left in place or replaced for a period of 2–7 days. Your physician will advise you to the timing of its removal or substitution. Take care to avoid disturbing the dressing while it is in place. Keep your head elevated. Don't sleep on your side.

Minor bleeding or oozing may occur. This is absolutely normal. Keep the area clean with a soft cloth. BE CAREFUL NOT TO PULL ANY STITCHES OR CRUSTS. You may keep clean, white towels around your neck to collect some of the oozing material.

Activity:

- Don't bend forward for the first 10 days.
- Don't carry any weight over 10 lb.
- Don't exercise for the first 10 days.
- Don't engage in sexual activities for 10 days.
- Don't drive for 10 days.
- Don't do any housework, cooking, etc. for 10 days.

- Don't dye or bleach hair for 30 days.
- Don't wax, have electrolysis, chemical or laser hair removal on face for 30 days.
- Don't wear contact lenses for at least 1 week after procedure.

You may read, talk, walk with moderation.

If you have had full-face resurfacing or perioral resurfacing only, prepare a liquid or semiliquid diet for at least 3–5 days. Make sure meals are well balanced.

Keep a humidifier near your face; avoid direct fans and heaters from your room.

Do not wash your hair until we give you permission.

Pain medication: You may experience a minimal discomfort that doesn't require pain medication; however, due to personal pain tolerance, some patients may request a pain medication prescription.

It is very important for your healing to surround yourself with positive people who understand as well as you do what you are going through. Don't forget that you should give yourself some time for healing.

Trust your doctor and trust the office staff. They are there to help you.

Do not miss your first postop appointment.

Home care instructions

Days 1–7 following laser surgery

1. Leave the dressing in place.
2. You probably will not require pain medication, but we will prescribe something if necessary.
3. Continue taking antiviral and antibiotic medication until we tell you to stop.
4. Apply to areas not covered by mask or dressing
   ( ) Eye ointment
   ( ) Postlaser balm
5. In the areas not covered by mask or dressing, a crust can begin to form over the treated areas. This should not be picked or scratched but should be gently removed with cleansing. DO NOT ALLOW CRUST TO FORM! It should be gently removed with repeated cleansing with one tablespoon of white vinegar to four glasses of water. It will help remove debris that may accumulate from the oozing of the treated skin. A soft cloth may be used.
6. If the perioral area has been resurfaced, a liquid diet or semisolid food is recommended.

Days 7–10 postop

1. Use postlaser cleanser
   ( )
2. Use postlaser balm
   ( )

Days 10–21 postop

- Discontinue antiviral medication
- Discontinue antibiotic medication

Topical treatment

AM
Cleanser
Postlaser balm
PM
Cleanser
Postlaser balm

Sun protection such as umbrella, hats, visors, and sunglasses, when outdoors. Don't stay near sunny windows. Skin is very sensitive.

Day 21

- Keep the AM/PM cleansing routine
- Lighter moisturizer: daily lotion with SPF-15
- Camouflage makeup
- Fade cream 4% (if there is any hyperpigmentation)

CHAPTER 16

Laser Facial Rejuvenation Complications: Diagnosis and Treatment

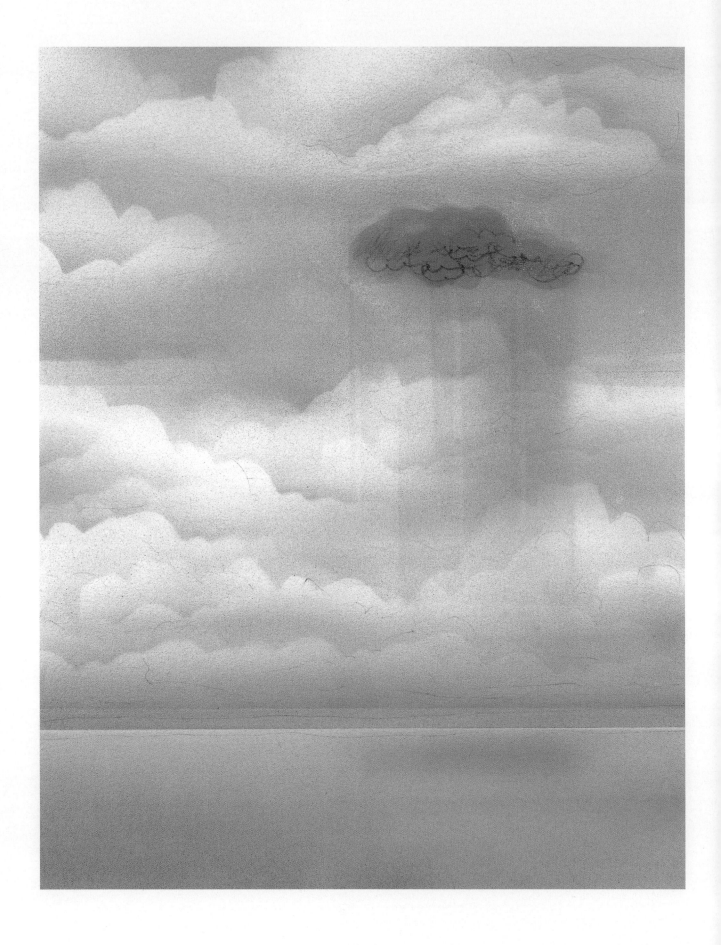

The bulk of our laser facial rejuvenation to this point has been performed with the carbon dioxide (CO_2) laser, most frequently with the UltraPulse CPG (computer pattern generator) (Coherent Medical, Palo Alto, CA). These are powerful instruments. Our best recommendations for the management of complications when using resurfacing techniques is to recognize where there is potential for complications to occur and then avoid these instances. Our most recent experience with the erbium:yttrium-aluminum-garnet (Er:YAG) laser has demonstrated its effectiveness and its great margin of safety when used cautiously, but the potential for complications exists nonetheless. Surgeons must understand the principles of these techniques and assimilate the experience of their mentors.

The potential complications of laser facial rejuvenation include infection, scarring, permanent dyspigmentation, prolonged erythema.

INFECTION

We have not had any patients with bacterial infections, but we recognize that they may occur and therefore begin intranasal mupirocin (Bactroban) 1 day before surgery and continue it until the patient is completely reepithelialized. As a rule, we do not use systemic antibiotics in New York but do use cephalexin (e.g., Keflex) 500 mg orally twice a day prophylactically, when performing this procedure in tropical environments; its use is continued until reepithelialization is complete.

Likewise, we do not treat with an antifungal agent prophylactically. If there is a postoperative white dusting of the face and delayed reepithelialization, we treat with fluconazole (Diflucan) 200 mg twice a day.

Herpes simplex infections are not uncommon. They most frequently occur if the patient has stopped taking the medication. Any patient complaining of postoperative pain is suspected of having a herpes simplex infection. Although we continue medicating our patients until reepithelialization is complete, on rare occasions, there may be a late recurrence of herpes infection in patients with a positive past history. Our drug of choice remains acyclovir (Zovirax) 200 mg orally four times a day. Many of our patients complain of gastrointestinal upsets when taking valacyclovir (Valtrex).

CICATRIZATION

We believe excessive cicatrization can be avoided by exerting caution when applying the CO_2 and Er:YAG lasers. We maintain the philosophy that more treatment can always be given at a later date—that it is better to undertreat than to overtreat. Adhering to safe settings and avoiding potential areas of trouble—the eyelid pretarsal areas, the lateral canthal angle, and the corners of the mouth—will decrease the likelihood of unacceptable results.

Local areas of hypertrophic scarring can first be massaged with betamethasone cream 0.1% to 0.5%. If there is no response in 1 week, intradermal triamcinolone acetonide (Kenalog) injections (diluted to 5 mg/mL) can be given in 0.1-mL amounts.

Mild to moderate cicatricial retraction of the lower lids can be corrected with recession of the lower lid retractors and lateral canthal suspension, while topical skin treatment is continued. In extreme cases, free-skin grafts may be necessary.

DYSPIGMENTATION

Postinflammatory hyperpigmentation is not uncommon and is transient. However, it can be exacerbated with sun exposure and by topical allergic reactions. Darkly pigmented patients who are subject to continued sun exposure after laser resurfacing will have a prolonged course of hyperpigmentation. After laser resurfacing, patients are exceptionally sensitive to topical agents. Previously well tolerated agents may now be markedly sensitizing. The use of creams or lotions not approved by the surgeon may subject the patient to a prolonged erythematous eruption with prolonged secondary dyspigmentation.

After the initial erythema is gone, topical bleaching agents can be started when hyperpigmentation is evident. Twice-daily applications can be reduced in frequency if superficial irritation is noted. Weekly glycolic acid peels can also accelerate fading. During this period of active treatment, application of a sun block is essential.

Bibliography

Adamson JE. Use of a muscle flap in lower blepharoplasty. *Plast Reconstr Surg* 1979;63:359.

Alster TS, Garg S. Treatment of facial rhytids with a high-energy pulsed CO_2 laser. *Plast Reconstr Surg* 1996;98:791–794.

Apfelberg DB. A critical appraisal of high-energy pulsed CO_2 laser resurfacing in acne scars. *Ann Plast Surg* 1997;38:95–199.

Aston SJ. Orbicularis oculi muscle flaps: a technique to reduce crow's-feet and lateral canthal skin folds. *Plast Reconstr Surg* 1980;65:206.

Aston SJ. Cosmetic surgery of the eyebrow and forehead. Presented at the 18th annual scientific symposium of the American Society of Ophthalmic Plastic and Reconstructive Surgery, Dallas, Texas, November 7, 1987.

Baker SS. Carbon dioxide laser upper lid blepharoplasty. *Am J Cosmet Surg* 1992;9:141–145.

Baker SS, Glaser DA. *Periorbital and facial laser applications.* St. Louis, MO: Medical Video Productions, 1996.

Baker SS, Muenzler WS, Small RG, Leonard JE. Carbon dioxide laser blepharoplasty. *Ophthalmology* 1984;91:238–244.

Baker SS, Muenzler WS, Small RG, et al. Carbon dioxide laser blepharoplasty. *Ophthalmology* 1984;91:243–283.

Baker TJ. Chemical face peeling and rhytidectomy. *Plast Reconstr Surg* 1962;29:199.

Bosniak S. *The video atlas of cosmetic blepharoplasty*, vol I. St. Louis, MO: Medical Video Productions, 1993.

Bosniak S, Cantisano-Zilkha M. *The video atlas of cosmetic blepharoplasty*, vol II. St. Louis, MO. Medical Video Productions, 1995.

Bosniak S, Cantisano-Zilkha M. Guide to ophthalmologists for patient selection and care in eyelid and facial rejuvenation. *J Brazil Soc Ophthalmol* 1997;56:899–904.

Castanares S. Classification of baggy eyelids deformity. *Plast Reconstr Surg* 1972;59:529.

Cohen IK, Peacock EE, Chvapil M. Zyderm. *Plast Reconstr Surg* 1984;73:857.

Courtiss EH. Selection of alternatives in esthetic blepharoplasty. *Clin Plast Surg* 1981;8:739–755.

David LM, Sanders G. CO_2 laser blepharoplasty: a comparison to cold steel and electrocautery. *J Dermatol Surg Oncol* 1987;13:110–114.

DeLustro F, Smith ST, Sundsmo J, Salem G, Kincaid S, Ellingsworth L. Reaction to injectable collagen: results in animal models and clinical use. *Plast Reconstr Surg* 1987;74:581–592.

Dupuis C, Rees, TD. Historical notes on blepharoplasty. *Plast Reconstr Surg* 1971;47:246.

Eaglstein WH, Davis SC, Mehle AL, Mertz PM. Optimal use of an occlusive dressing to enhance healing: effect of delayed application and early removal on wound healing. *Arch Dermatol* 1988;124:392.

Ellenbogen R. Trancoronal eyebrow lift with concomitant blepharoplasty. *Plast Reconstr Surg* 1983;71:490–499.

Feist DR, Surcliffe RT, Baylis HI. The coronal brow lift. *Am J Ophthalmol* 1983;96:751.

Fernandez LR. The double eyelid operation in the Oriental of Hawaii. *Plast Reconstr Surg* 1960;25:257.

Fisher JC. Discussion of reaction of injectable collagen: result in animal models and clinical use. *Plast Reconstr Surg* 1987;79:593.

Fitzpatrick RE, Goldman MP. Advances in carbon dioxide laser surgery. *Clin Dermatol* 1995;13:35–47.

Fitzpatrick RE, Goldman MP, Satur MN, Tope WD. Pulsed CO_2 laser resurfacing of photodamaged facial skin. *Arch Dermatol* 1996;132:395–402.

Flowers RS. Anchor blepharoplasty. *Transactions of the International Congress of Plastic Surgeons.* Paris: Masson, 1976;135–137.

Flowers RS. Tear trough implants for correction of tear trough deformity. *Clin Plast Surg* 1993;20:403.

Fodor PB. Endoscopic plastic surgery, a new milestone in plastic surgery [Editorial]. *Aesthetic Plast Surg* 1994;18:31.

Furnas DW. Festoons of orbicularis muscle as a cause of baggy eyelids. *Plast Reconstr Surg* 1978;61:531.

Goldbaum AM, Woog JJ. The CO_2 laser in oculoplastic surgery. *Surv Ophthalmol* 1997;42:255–267.

Hamra ST. *Composite rhytidectomy.* St. Louis, MO: Quality Medical Publishing, 1993.

Hisatomi C, Fujino T. Anatomical considerations concerning blepharoplasty in the Oriental patient. In: Bosniak S, ed. *Advances in ophthalmic plastic and reconstructive surgery, vol II: the aging face.* Elmsford, NY: Pergamon Press, 1982;151–161.

Hueston JT, Heinze JB. Successful early relief of blindness occurring after blepharoplasty. *Plast Reconstr Surg* 1972;53:588.

Hunter D, Frumkin A. Adverse reactions to vitamin E and aloe vera preparations after dermabrasion and chemical peel. *Cutis* 1991;47:193.

Isse N. The endoscopic forehead lift. Presented at the interdisciplinary facial plastic surgery symposium, Santa Barbara, California, November 12, 1995.

Johnson CC. Epiblepharon. *Am J Ophthalmol* 1968;66:1172–1175.

Johnson CC. Epicanthus and epiblepharon. *Arch Ophthalmol* 1978;96:1030–1033.

Katzen LB, Karvelis JJ. Anesthesia, analgesia, amnesia. In: Putterman A, ed. *Cosmetic oculoplastic surgery.* New York: Grune & Stratton, 1982;90–97.

Kaufmann R, Hibst R. Pulsed erbium YAG laser ablation in cutaneous surgery. *Lasers Surg Med* 1996;19:324–330.

Kaye BL. The forehead lift: a useful adjunct to face lift and blepharoplasty. *Plast Reconstr Surg* 1977;60:161.

Keller GS. Transblepharoplasty brow suspension with the KTP laser. *Int J Aesthetic Restor Surg* 1993;1:101–105.

Kligman AM, Grove GL, Hrose R, et al. Topical tretinoin for photoaged skin. *J Am Acad Dermatol* 1986;15:836–859.

Knapp TR, Kaplan EN, Daniels JR. Injectable collagen for soft tissue augmentation. *Plast Reconstr Surg* 1977;60:30–45.

Kohn R, Romano PE. Blepharoptosis, blepharophimosis, epicanthus inversus and telecanthus: a syndrome with no name. *Am J Ophthalmol* 72;1971:625–632.

Lemke BN, Stasior OG. The anatomy of eyebrow ptosis. *Arch Ophthalmol* 1982;100:981.

Lemke BN, Stasior OG. Eyebrow considerations in blepharoptosis. In: Bosniak S, ed. *Advances in ophthalmic plastic and reconstructive surgery, vol I: ptosis.* Elmsford, NY: Pergamon Press, 1983;55–67.

Lemke BN, Stasior OG. Eyebrow incision making. In: Bosniak S, ed. *Advances in ophthalmic plastic and reconstructive surgery, vol II: the aging face.* Elmsford, NY: Pergamon Press, 1983;19–23.

Litton C. Observation after chemosurgery of the face. *Plast Reconstr Surg* 1963;32:544–556.

Lynch S. Hypnosis, amnesia, anesthesia. In: Rees TD, Woodsmith D, eds. *Cosmetic facial surgery*. Philadelphia: WB Saunders, 1973;34–43.

Millard DR. Oriental peregrinations. *Plast Reconstr Surg* 1955;16:337.

Millard DR Jr. The Oriental eyelid and its surgical revision. *Am J Ophthalmol* 1964;57:646–649.

Morax S. The use of Gore-Tex in recession of upper lid retractors. Presented at the annual meeting of the European Society of Ophthalmic Plastic and Reconstructive Surgery, Capri, Italy, 1987.

Morrow DM, Morrow LB. CO_2 laser blepharoplasty: a comparison with cold-steel surgery. *J Dermatol Surg Oncol* 1992;18:307–313.

Mosher DB, Fitzpatrick TB, Hori Y, Ortonne JP. Disorders of melanocytes. In: Fitzpatrick TB, ed. *Dermatology in general medicine*, 4th ed. New York: McGraw-Hill, 1993;903–995.

Owsley JQ. Lifting the malar fat pad for correction of prominent nasolabial folds. *Plast Reconstr Surg* 1993;91:463.

Pang HS. Surgical formation of the upper lid fold. *Arch Ophthalmol* 1961;65:783.

Ramirez OM. Endoscopic full facelift. *Aesthetic Plast Surg* 1994;18:363.

Ramirez OM. Endoscopic options in facial rejuvenation: an overview. *Aesthetic Plast Surg* 1994;18:141–147.

Ramirez OM. Endoscopically assisted biplanar forehead left. *Plast Reconstr Surg* 1995;97:323–333.

Ramirez OM, Mailard GF, Musolas A. The extended subperiosteal facelift: a definitive soft tissue remodeling for facial rejuvenation. *Plast Reconstr Surg* 1991;88:227.

Rees TD. Technical considerations in blepharoplasty and rhytidectomy. *Transactions of the Fifth International Congress of Plastic and Reconstructive Surgery, Australia, 1971*. Sidney: Butterworth, 1971;1067.

Rees TD. *Aesthetic plastic surgery*, vol II. Philadelphia: WB Saunders, 1980.

Rees TD, Dupois C. Cosmetic blepharoplasty in the older age group. *Ophthalmol Surg* 1970;1:30.

Rees TD, Dupois C. Baggy eyelids in young adults. *Plast Reconstr* Surg 1969;43:381.

Riefrohl R. The forehead-brow lift. *Ann Plast Surg* 1982;8:55.

Roberts TL, Lettieri JT, Ellis LB. CO_2 laser resurfacing: recognizing and minimizing complications. *Aesthetic Surg Q* 1996;16:142.

Rosenberg GT, Gregory RO. Lasers in aesthetic surgery. *Clin Plast Surg* 1996;23:29–48.

Rubin MG. *Manual of chemical peels*. Philadelphia: JB Lippincott Co, 1995.

Sachs ME, Bosniak SL, Leinhardt RR. Procedural options in cosmetic blepharoplasty. In: Bosniak S, ed. *Advances in ophthalmic plastic and reconstructive surgery, vol II: the aging face*. Elmsford, NY: Pergamon Press, 1983;55–74.

Sartin J. Pre- and postoperative facial care: restoring the aging face and ameliorating the effects of aging. In: Bosniak S, ed. *Advances in ophthalmic plastic and reconstructive surgery, vol II: the aging face*. Elmsford, NY: Pergamon Press, 1983;217–219.

Sasaki G. Brow ptosis. In: Sasaki G, ed. *Endoscopic, aesthetic, and reconstructive surgery*. Philadelphia: Lippincott–Raven Publishers, 1996;19–28.

Sayoc BT. Plastic construction of the superior palpebral fold. *Am J Ophthalmol* 1954;38:556.

Seckel BR. *Aesthetic laser surgery*. Boston: Little, Brown and Company, 1995.

Sheen JH. A change in the technique of supratarsal fixation in upper blepharoplasty. *Plast Reconstr Surg* 1977;59:836.

Small RG. Periosteal fixation in reconstructive blepharoplasty. In: Bosniak S, ed. *Advances in ophthalmic plastic and reconstructive surgery, vol II: the aging face*. Elmsford, NY: Pergamon Press, 1983;89–99.

Smith BC, Bosniak S. Reconstructing the supratarsal crease. In: Bosniak S, ed. *Advances in ophthalmic plastic and reconstructive surgery, vol I: ptosis*. Elmsford, NY: Pergamon Press, 1981;75–87.

Smith BC, Nesi F. Complications of cosmetic blepharoplasty. *Trans Amer Acad Ophthalmol* 1978;85:726–729.

Stasior OG, Lemke BN. The posterior eyebrow fixation. In: Bosniak S, ed. *Advances in ophthalmic plastic and reconstructive surgery, vol II: the aging face*. Elmsford, NY: Pergamon Press, 1983;193–197.

Steaman S, Romonitch J. Implantation of collagen for depressed scars. *J Dermatol Surg Oncol* 1980;62:499.

Stuzin JM, Baker TJ, Baker TM, Kligman AM. Histologic effects of the high-energy pulsed CO_2 laser on photoaged skin. *Plast Reconstr Surg* 1997;99:2036–2050.

Tabbal N. Special techniques in cosmetic surgery. In: Smith B, Della Rocca RC, Nesi FA, Lisman RD, eds. *Ophthalmic plastic and reconstructive surgery*. St. Louis, MO: CV Mosby Co, 1987;721–731.

Trelles MA, Sanchez J, Sala P, et al. Surgical removal of lower eyelid fat using the carbon dioxide laser. *Am J Cosmet Surg* 1992;9:149–152.

Vasconez LO, Core GB, Gamboa-Bobadilla M, et al. Endoscopic techniques in coronal brow lifting. *Plast Reconstr Surg* 1994;94:788–793.

Vinas JX, Caviglia C, Cortinas JL. Forehead rhytidoplasty and brow lifting. *Plast Reconstr Surg* 1976;57:455.

Weinstein C, Alster TS. Skin resurfacing with high-energy, pulsed carbon dioxide lasers. In: Alster TS, Apfelberg DG, eds. *Cosmetic laser surgery*. New York: John Wiley and Sons, 1996;9–27.

Weinstein C, Ramirez OM, Pozner JN. Postoperative care following CO_2 laser resurfacing: avoiding pitfalls. *Plast Reconstr Surg* 1997;100:1855–1866.

Weiss JS, Ellis CN, Headington JT, Tincoff T, Hamiltion TA, Voorhess JJ. Topical tretinoin improves photoaged skin: a double-blind vehicle-controlled study. *JAMA* 1988;259:527–532.

Subject Index

Page numbers followed by f indicate figures; page numbers followed by t indicate tables.